For my mother and father

Acknowledgements

With many thanks to all who made this book possible. Thank you to my daughter, Zara Light for her excellent editing. Thank you to Betsy Carver for her expert assistance in layout.

This publication contains the opinions and ideas of the author. It is intended to provide helpful and informative material on the subjects addressed in this publication. It is sold with the understanding that the author and publisher are not engaged in rendering medical, health, psychological, or any other kind of personal professional services in the book. The nutrition advice is intended to support not to take the place of any medical treatment.

The author and publisher specifically disclaim all responsibility for any liability, loss, or risk, personal or otherwise, that is incurred as a consequence, directly or indirectly, of the use and application of any of the contents of this book.

The Library of Congress Cataloging-in-Publication Data is available.
ISBN-978-0-395-97789-7

The Cancer Nutrition Center Handbook

An Essential Guide for Cancer Patients and their Families

Carolyn Katzin, MSPH, CNS

CfK
Los Angeles, CA

CONTENTS

INTRODUCTION

In 1986, I began working with participants (those who had been diagnosed with cancer but were not defined by that diagnosis) at The Wellness Community in the Little Yellow House in Santa Monica. Each Friday, I would prepare lunch and share why food was especially important for them. I explained how eating well would improve their resilience and help them to face the challenges that lay ahead. The late Harold Benjamin founded The Wellness Community after his wife was diagnosed with breast cancer. He was a wonderful mentor and inspiration to me and thousands of other people with his Patient Active concept. Soon I was recruited as a volunteer for the American Cancer Society and so began an amazing journey of learning and teaching. Over the past twenty years, my nutrition practice has specialized in assisting those faced with cancer. I have been fortunate enough to work with thousands of people, helping them to optimize their diet and include effective but safe dietary supplements. In my experience, good nutrition is empowering and may even be healing.

I developed a nutrition guide for participants of The Wellness Community and have published two earlier editions which have been for sale on my website since 1997. This guide is a living document and I owe much to the input I have received from so many cancer patients and their loved ones. I thank them all from the bottom of my heart.

The information in this handbook is arranged to assist those newly diagnosed, those undergoing treatment and for survivors and all of us who wish to be in optimal health. The Cycle of Nutrition and Cancer describes how during active treatment it is often difficult to eat a healthy diet due to poor appetite, fatigue and also because such a diet is usually high in dietary fiber and may take a lot of effort to chew. In my opinion, right after diagnosis the most important thing to do is to maintain a healthy weight and stay strong. This may mean eating foods that are higher in healthy oils or fats and selecting foods that are easy to digest. The cycle can be used as a map to guide you; when you are well you should eat as healthily as you can. During treatment, you need to consume sufficient calories to keep up your strength. I call this the Expedient Diet. However, as the acute treatment time is usually short, this is a time to choose tasty foods you like and want to eat above all. Later on, you can make up for any possible nutritional imbalances by eating especially beneficial foods and supplements in, what I term, the Regenerative phase of the cycle. Many people have thanked me for providing this charted course of nutrition as it has helped them to fend off well-meaning but often bossy or intrusive dietary suggestions from friends and family. You can simply tell them about the Cycle of Nutrition for Cancer Patients and that you are in your Expedient Diet phase when you reach for the only thing you fancy, even if it may not be a healthy item in isolation.

My desire is that this book and the recipes at the end will assist you and your family in making this journey a little easier.

Carolyn Katzin
Los Angeles, June, 2006

NUTRITION GUIDELINES for everyone

The National Cancer Institute and the American Cancer Society estimate that 35% of all cancers are linked to diet. For women, this is as high as ONE HALF of all cancers. Physical activity is also vitally important and when combined with a healthy diet, they both provide the best opportunity for staying healthy. Fresh, wholesome food is crucial for a healthy immune system.

1. Choose at least five servings (or about 1 ½ pounds) of fruits and vegetables each day. Many studies show a decreased risk of lung, prostate, bladder, esophageal and stomach cancers with plenty of fruits and vegetables in the diet. The average American consumes only three servings and this may include tomato ketchup and French fries! Dark green, yellow and orange types of vegetables are the richest in protective botanical factors also called phytonutrients. Blueberries and dark red grapes are also rich in antioxidants, anticarcinogens and anti-inflammatory botanical factors. I call these the three A's. Choose most of the foods you eat from plant sources. Choose whole grains as opposed to refined or processed ones as they have more B vitamins, zinc, magnesium and other important nutrients. Choose beans often as an alternative to meat. Select organically grown produce whenever you can.

2. Limit your intake of high fat foods, particularly from animal sources. High fat diets have been associated with an increase in the risk of cancers of the colon and rectum, prostate and endometrium. The association with breast cancer is weaker. Choose foods low in animal fat by replacing fat-rich foods with fruits, vegetables, grains and beans. Eat smaller portions and select non-fat or low-fat (1%) dairy products. When eating meat select lean cuts and bake or broil rather than fry meat, seafood and poultry. Healthy oils do not need to be restricted; these include oily fish, olives, avocado, nuts and seeds. These are beneficial.

3. Be physically active: achieve and maintain a healthy weight. Physical activity can help to protect against some cancers and assist in recovery. At least thirty minutes of moderate activity on most days of the week is recommended for well being. Physical activity stimulates bowel health and may play a part in normalizing hormone levels and reducing prostate and breast cancer risks. Recent studies have suggested a protection from skin cancer which may also be related to vitamin D due to the action of sunlight on the skin.

4. Limit consumption of alcoholic beverages, if you drink at all. In countries where alcohol consumption is high (more than two drinks a day) oral and esophageal cancers are more common. There is a more than additive effect with smoking. Moderate intakes of wine or beer with food are associated with improved cardiovascular health and add to the enjoyment of a meal. Larger amounts may provide calories at the expense of more nutrient rich and cancer protective foods and are not recommended. The American Cancer Society recommends no alcohol at all if you have a family history of breast cancer.

Remember that moderation and variety are the keys to a healthy diet and lifestyle.

EATING TO REDUCE YOUR RISK OF CANCER

◆ Eat fresh fruit and a salad every day. Use olive oil and lemon juice or balsamic vinegar as a salad dressing. Sprinkle a few pine nuts (pignolas), walnuts or almonds on top for healthy omega-3 fatty acids, B vitamins and dietary fiber. Hard boiled egg white increases the protein.
◆ Eat at least 5 servings of fruits and vegetables each day. For most people this means simply adding one more serving. 8-10 servings are even better for you as they are rich in the three A's Antioxidants, Anticarcinogens and Anti-inflammatories.
◆ Half a cup of berries (fresh or frozen) has as much cancer-fighting antioxidant activity as 5 servings of most other fruits and vegetables.
◆ Eat high fiber, folate rich beans and peas 3 or more times a week. Vary your types of beans: black, Mung, garbanzo, kidney, soy, green beans and peas.
◆ Wash fruits and vegetables well and eat with the skin on whenever possible. The skin and just under the skin are where most of the nutrients and fiber are.
◆ Cabbage (all types), broccoli, Brussels sprouts, bok choy and other cruciferous vegetables are particularly rich in cancer fighting phytonutrients or botanical factors.
◆ Try tofu, soy milk and cheese, and other soy foods for a variety of cancer fighting factors (restrict edamame if you have estrogen receptor positive breast cancer).
◆ Add half a cup of wheat germ to your breakfast cereals for added B vitamins, vitamin E and dietary fiber.
◆ Use instant oatmeal in meat loaf recipes for added fiber.
◆ Include fresh fruit or whole juices often. If drinking juices make sure they are 100% juice as some labels can be misleading.
◆ Include spinach often. It is rich in cancer fighting nutrients. Wash well and eat small, fresh leaves if possible or lightly steamed.
◆ Include watercress often. It is rich in beta carotene and other phytonutrients.
◆ Use garlic when cooking. Garlic was mentioned by Hippocrates 2500 years ago as a cancer fighting food.
◆ When using lemons and limes, remember to twist the zest for the essential oils in the rind. These are particularly good cancer fighters.
◆ Eat cantaloupe, pomegranates, blueberries, apricots, spinach and carrots often for beta carotene and other cancer fighting phytonutrients.
◆ Eat watermelon, pink grapefruit, tomato paste in your sauce and fresh tomatoes often for lycopene and other cancer fighting phytonutrients.
◆ Eat green, red and yellow bell peppers often for Vitamin C and other cancer fighting nutrients. Slice and add to salads or chop finely into other dishes.
◆ Always include lettuce and tomato in your sandwiches. If you like, add peppers and onions too.
◆ Eat fish often. Choose wild salmon often. Tuna, halibut, herrings or sardines are all good choices. Remember to vary your types of fresh fish. Many people who eat fish regularly have a reduced risk of heart disease, stroke and possibly some forms of cancer too.
◆ Eat red grapes and drink red grape juice or small quantities of red wine (unless you have breast cancer in the family when the American Cancer Society suggests you do not drink alcohol at all). Red grapes contain a cancer fighting nutrient resveratrol as well as other healthful phytonutrients.

Standard Serving Sizes

- Fruits
  - 1 medium apple, banana, orange
  - Half a cup of chopped, cooked or canned fruit
  - 3/4 cup of 100% fruit juice
- Vegetables
  - 1 cup of raw vegetables
  - Half a cup of cooked vegetables
  - Half a cup of chopped raw vegetables
  - 3/4 cup vegetable juice
- Grains
  - 1 slice bread
  - 1 ounce ready-to-eat cereal
  - Half a cup of cooked cereal, rice, pasta
- Beans and nuts
  - Half a cup cooked beans
  - 2 tablespoons peanut butter
  - 1/3 cup nuts (what fits in the palm of your hand)
- Dairy foods and eggs
  - 1 cup milk or yogurt
  - One and a half ounces of natural cheese
  - 2 ounces of processed cheese
- Meat and fish
  - 2-3 ounces (size and weight of a pack of cards)
  - Lean meat, poultry and fish

HEALTHY BODY WEIGHT

Increasing evidence suggests that maintaining a healthy body weight is very important to your quality of life. Body Mass Index (BMI) is often used as a general guide. You can check yours by going to the American Cancer Society website at www.cancer.org. BMI is the ratio of your height to your weight, and ideally, should be between 19 and 24.9. Over 25 is considered overweight and over 30 is considered obese. A pear rather than an apple shape is also linked to health but this tends to be genetic and difficult to alter. A healthy waist size is considered to be 40 inches or under for men (usually related to a pant size two inches smaller) and 35 inches or under for women. Central adiposity or belly fat is associated with higher risks of inflammation and this may be particularly important if you have been diagnosed with cancer. Belly fat is responsive to exercise especially core type such as yoga or Pilates.

Try marking a tape measure with your goal waist measurement and check regularly. Rapid weight change should be brought to the attention of your health professional (+/- 5 lbs. a week).

THREE STAGES IN THE CYCLE OF NUTRITION AND CANCER

1. Preventive Nutrition (when you feel well)
   ◆ Fats or oils from fish, nuts and seeds need not be restricted. Saturated fats from meats, dairy products or hydrogenated oils should be restricted to less than 10% of total energy intake.
   ◆ Rich in foods from plant sources such as whole grains, beans, starchy root vegetables, nuts, green, leafy vegetables and darkly pigmented fruits.
   ◆ Reasonable in protein: two servings daily (about the size of a deck of cards) of fish, lean meat, poultry or one cup of mixed beans and rice.
   ◆ Plenty of antioxidants and phytonutrients or botanical factors found in whole grains, beans, vegetables and many fruits. Dark colored items are richest sources. Eat some frequently.
   ◆ Moderate quantities overall. Stay active to maintain a steady weight.
   ◆ Wide variety of foods, especially seasonal fruits and vegetables. Eat a minimum of 5 servings each day, 8-10 servings are recommended.
2. During Treatment (Expedient Diet)
   ◆ Frequent, easily-digested, small meals of sufficient energy to maintain body weight.
   ◆ Stay as active as possible. Try walking, stretching, yoga and stress reducing types of activities.
   ◆ One more serving per day of protein; use protein powder for smoothies or include hard boiled eggs on salads or add egg whites, more fish and poultry at meal times.
   ◆ Few dairy products due to possible lactose-intolerance which may develop; symptoms include abdominal discomfort and diarrhea. Live culture yogurt or hard cheese is usually okay.
   ◆ Avoid gas-producing foods such as insufficiently cooked beans or excessive amounts of the cabbage family. Use digestive enzymes to reduce gas and bloating.
   ◆ Avoid highly spiced foods, unless they agree with you.
   ◆ Be especially vigilant with food safety.
   ◆ Avoid more than RDA's of antioxidant supplements.
3. Regenerative Nutrition (as you recover and transition back to Preventive (Survivorship)
   ◆ As with Preventive Nutrition but with a special focus on the nutrients needed for regenerating the immune system, for instance Vitamins B, C, E, selenium and zinc. Try adding a tablespoon of wheat or rice germ to your morning cereal.
   ◆ Be physically active, introducing more varieties and intensity of exercise as you feel better.
   ◆ At least 10 servings of fruits and vegetables each day. Try 100% fruit or vegetable juices but remember to wash all produce well. Food safety is still a vitally important aspect of your recovery.
   ◆ Reintroduce milk and lactose containing dairy products slowly.
   ◆ Include a daily antioxidant rich multivitamin and mineral supplement.

PERSONALIZED NUTRITION

In 2001, the first draft of the human genome was completed and now personalized nutrition has become a reality. By the time you read this you may already have had your DNA analyzed to learn how fast you metabolize certain medications (www.genelex.com offers an excellent range of these pharmacogenomic tests). If you are taking more than three medications on a regular basis I encourage you to learn more about your liver enzyme profiles.

In addition to how efficiently your body metabolizes medications and herbs you may also wish to learn more about how you handle the approximately 23,000 different food components you may be exposed to on any typical day. This is called a nutrigenomic test and I offer this at my website www.thednadiet.com. Common variations in our molecular identity or genetic code occur very frequently and offer insights into how well you may handle certain foods. For instance, you may have variations that affect your insulin sensitivity. Once you know this you can choose low glycemic foods (those that release sugar slowly into your blood stream), eat small, frequent meals and choose healthy oils which also slow down stomach emptying.

For most people the Mediterranean Diet is recommended as being healthiest; it is rich in colorful vegetables and fruits especially tomatoes and citrus fruits. Fish is eaten frequently (at least twice a week) and red meat is limited. Olives, almonds, pistachios and other sources of healthy oils are eaten frequently and salads are dressed with extra virgin olive oil. Beans (fava, garbanzo, green beans, etc.) are also eaten frequently providing B vitamins and dietary fiber. Most of the recipes in this book are based on the Mediterranean Diet and provide colorful botanical benefits.

Red grapes and red wine are rich in resveratrol which is a powerful antioxidant. Many people enjoy a glass of red wine or red grape juice with their meal. I suggest selecting organic wines wherever possible. Dark chocolate is another excellent source of resveratrol and other antioxidants. Again, organic is best.

NUTRITION DURING TREATMENT

If you have been diagnosed with cancer, eating well is one of the most important things for you to consider as part of your whole treatment regimen. A simple rule of thumb is to maintain a steady body weight throughout treatment. This means neither gaining too much, nor losing too much weight (fluctuations of more than 5lbs per week for an average sized adult). If you are overweight at the beginning of treatment it is safe to lose about a pound a week but this probably isn't the time to embark on a weight loss diet.

Preparing for Treatment:

Surgery: Eat a low fat (less than 25% of calories), high protein diet of two or three protein rich foods such as fish, eggs, chicken or lean meat; beans and rice if vegetarian. Supplement with a multivitamin and mineral supplement containing DAILY VALUE amounts. An additional supplement containing 500 mg vitamin C with bioflavonoids taken every 8 hours for 2 days before surgery and for a week afterwards may be beneficial to healing. Stop all supplements of vitamins E and K, evening primrose, borage or fish oils one week before surgery as these may cause thinning of the blood. Do not take any herbs without informing your medical team as they may interfere with other medications. Avoid grapefruit juice as this may affect liver enzyme clearance of some medications.

Radiation: Usual preventive nutrition diet but no supplements beyond usual RDA level multivitamin of vitamin C or E.

Chemotherapy: Eat a low fat, high carbohydrate diet the day before chemotherapy. No supplements on day of treatment.

During Treatment:

Surgery: According to your medical professionals' protocols.

Radiation: Extra carbohydrate calories: try green tea or Siberian ginseng for energy.

Chemotherapy: Avoid eating your favorite foods within 24 hours of treatment to avoid negative associations with them at a later time. Eat a low fat (less than 3 tablespoons or 40 grams total fat or oil per day), high complex carbohydrate diet. Most of your energy should come from whole grain breads, cereals, beans, fruits and vegetables with an additional serving of protein. White meat chicken, fish and eggs are easy to digest. Protein powder based smoothies are also good. Avoid more than 100% Daily Value of antioxidant supplements as these may interfere with the clearance of the chemotherapy medications.

After Treatment:

Surgery: High protein diet; three servings daily of lean meat, poultry, fish or eggs or add in a protein smoothie. Regular supplements as above. Include an antioxidant supplement.

Radiation: High protein and energy diet. Lactose-free and relatively low in simple sugars (sucrose, lactose or honey) to avoid intestinal discomfort or bloating.

Chemotherapy: See next section for details of specific drug/nutrient interactions.

NUTRITION AND CHEMOTHERAPY

General Nutritional Advice

- Drink plenty of fluids - at least two liters total, with most of it coming from clear liquids such as water, apple juice, clear broths or Jell-o®. Avoid caffeine containing liquids such as tea, coffee and colas as these are dehydrating.
- Eat small quantities of food rather than large meals for easier digestion.
- Eat crackers, Melba toast, pasta and baked potatoes if you feel nauseated.
- Use the concept of the Expedient Diet and make up for eating less healthily, if needed, when you feel stronger.
- Eat avocado often as it is an excellent source of calories, essential fatty acids, potassium and glutathione, unless contraindicated (if on Procarbazine or other medication requiring a low tyramine diet).

Some Drug-Specific Nutritional Advice

Abraxane, Paclitaxel	Avoid caffeine, avoid grapefruit juice.
Accutane, Isoretinoin	Avoid alcohol; avoid sugar; eat low saturated animal fat diet; drink plenty of fluids.
Alimta, Pemetrexed	Vitamin B-12 and folate may be given. Avoid caffeine and alcohol.
Asparaginase, Elspar	Drink extra fluids; consume extra calories.
Bleomycin, Blenoxane	Bland foods.
Busulfan, Myleran	Drink extra fluids; eat foods rich in B vitamins.
Camptosar, Irinotecan	Drink extra fluids. Small, frequent bland meals.
Carmustine, BiCNU	Bland foods; avocado.
Chlorambucil, Leukeran	Drink extra fluids; bland foods; avocado.
Cisplatin and Carboplatin	Avoid purine rich foods (liver, caviar, sardines, anchovies) Eat plenty of magnesium, potassium and zinc rich foods (whole grains, nuts). Drink extra fluids.
Cladribine, 2-CdA, Leustatin	Drink extra fluids.
Cyclophosmide, Cytoxan	Drink extra fluids; don't cut back on salt or sodium containing foods;

	avoid alcohol; eat bland and low fat foods.
Cytarabine, Ara-C, Cytosar-U	Drink extra fluids; bland foods; avocado.
Dacarbazine,DITC-Dome	Drink extra fluids; bland foods; avocado.
Daunorubicin, Cerubine	Drink extra fluids; eat foods rich in B vitamins, particularly riboflavin (milk, lean meat, egg yolks, wheat germ).
Doxorubicin, Adriamycin	Drink extra fluids; eat foods rich in B vitamins particularly riboflavin.
Eloxatin, Oxaliplatin	Drink extra fluids.
Epirubicin chloride	Drink extra fluids (urine may turn pink).
Erbitux, Cetuximab	Eat magnesium, calcium and potassium rich foods. Avoid caffeine.
Etoposide, VePesid, VP-16	Bland foods; avocado.
5-Fluorouracil, Adrucil	Drink extra fluids; eat foods rich in B vitamins.
Fludarabine, Fludara-IV	Drink extra fluids.
Gleevec, imatinib mesylate	Low sodium. Avoid grapefruit juice. Take with food.
Hydroxyurea, Hydrea	Drink extra fluids.
Idarubicin, Idamycin	Drink extra fluids.
Ifosfamide, Ifex	Drink extra fluids.
Interferon, Intron, Roferon	Drink extra fluids; bland diet; avocado.
Idarubicin, Idamycin	Drink extra fluids.
Ifosfamide, Ifex	Drink extra fluids.
Irinotecan, Campto	Drink extra fluids. Small, frequent bland meals.
Lomustine, CeeNU	Bland foods; avocado.
Mechlorethamine, Mustargen	Drink extra fluids; restrict simple sugars.
Melphalan, Alkeran	Drink extra fluids.
Mercaptopurine, Purinethol	Drink extra fluids; avoid alcohol; avoid foods rich in purines (anchovies kidneys, liver, meat extracts, sardines, beans and lentils) Eat foods rich in B vitamins like wheat germ.
Methotrexate, Mexate	Drink extra fluids; avoid alcohol; bland diet; eat foods that produce an alkaline urine to assist excretion (almonds, milk, fruits and vegetables, except cranberries, plums, corn and lentils).
Mitomycin, Mutamycin	Drink extra fluids; bland diet; avocado; eat foods rich in folate (green, leafy vegetables, citrus fruits) and foods rich in calcium (dairy foods, broccoli).
Mitoxantrone, Novantrone	Drink extra fluids (discolored urine).
Pentostatin, Nipent	Bland foods; avocado.
Procarbazine, Matulane	Avoid tyramine containing foods (aged cheeses, yogurt, raisins, eggplant canned figs, salami, sour cream, avocados, bananas, soy sauce, lima beans, tenderized meats, etc. - ask for a list from your doctor) Maintain tyramine free diet for 14 days after treatment ceases; no alcohol.
Tamoxifen, Nolvadex	Avoid high fat foods; exercise regularly to minimize possible weight gain side effect; eat foods rich in calcium and magnesium (dairy foods, broccoli, nuts and seeds).
Taxol and Taxotere	Drink extra fluids.
Thalidomide, Thalomid	Avoid alcohol
6-Thioguanine, Tabloid	High fiber diet
Vinblastine, Velban	Drink extra fluids

Vincristine, Oncovin	Drink extra fluids; bland diet; avocado

Drugs often prescribed with Chemotherapy

Dexamethasone, Decadron	Low salt, high potassium diet (avocado, bananas, citrus fruits, most vegetables especially mushrooms)
Prednisone, Deltasone	Low sugar diet; no alcohol
Meticorten, Orasen	Low salt, high potassium diet; no alcohol
Megesterol, Megace	Low salt
Mesna, Mesnex	Plenty of fluids

If your oncologist is using combinations of the above medications modify the advice so that you retain the most important parts. Remember to ask about nutrition; request a consultation with a Medical Nutrition Therapist (a registered dietitian or other qualified nutritionist).

Here is an example of dietary advice for a combination regimen:

CMF Avoid fatty foods. Eat small quantities of bland flavors. Avoid alcohol, highly spiced foods or very acidic foods (cranberries, pineapple, lemons etc.). Focus on vegetables, lean meats moistened in liquids such as stews, casseroles or in soups. Increase fiber with whole grain breakfast cereals.

Many chemotherapy regimens affect your blood cell count. A nutritional supplement that is often described as hematinic, or blood building, may be valuable. Check with your oncologist before taking such a supplement in case it interferes with the chemotherapy. If you are prescribed a medication that stimulates new blood cell formation, include an extra serving of protein to get the optimal benefit. Remember to keep your health care team informed of all and any nutritional supplements (including herbal teas, fortified products and other functional foods).

RADIATION TREATMENT AND NUTRITION

Radiation can affect your taste buds so that food may taste bitter or you may have a metallic taste in your mouth. Some people find using non-metal utensils helpful. Try marinating meats for better flavor. Cold foods may be more palatable than hot but avoid extreme temperatures as your nerve endings may be compromised. Use herbs such as thyme, oregano, tarragon, mint and basil for added flavor. Try adding sauces such as apple sauce, yogurt dressings, mayonnaise and salad dressings to make food easier to chew. Snack on protein powder (whey, rice or soy) milk shakes. Ensure or other canned elemental diets are also useful standbys. Ask your health care professional or dietitian about products suitable for radiation enteritis or other chronic diarrhea situations. Examples include Resource Plus, Prosure, Vivonex and Peptamen. Radiation treatment should not be combined with high dose supplements of antioxidants (beta carotene, vitamins C and E or glutathione). The amounts found in a normal mixed diet will not interfere with treatment. To counteract gastrointestinal problems avoid milk and milk products as lactose intolerance may develop. Yogurt which uses a live culture may be tolerated well. You can use Lactaid milk and Lactaid drops to minimize discomfort with dairy products. Ensure and similar meal replacement drinks are lactose free.

SOME SUPPLEMENTS AND HELPFUL FOODS

Alpha Lipoic Acid	An important antioxidant involved in detoxification
Coenzyme Q10	Another antioxidant that may be beneficial during treatment
Garlic	Allicin (allythio sulfinic allyl ester) is a weak anti-cancer agent found in garlic. Recognized as early as 1550 BC as a treatment for cancer.
Papaya, Pineapple	Many tropical fruits contain natural enzymes that may be beneficial during treatment as well as preventively. Guava, noni and mangosteen also are good.
Green Tea	Contains protective botanical factors (catechins, polyphenols). Drink some daily.
Milk Thistle	This herb may assist in detoxification and general support of the liver detoxification enzyme systems. May be useful after chemotherapy. Also called Silymarin.
N-Acetyl Cysteine	Similar to alpha lipoic acid (see above), this is important in maintaining healthy liver and other tissue detoxification enzyme processes. Also called NAC.

Always consult with your physician before taking any nutritional supplements and inform all health care professionals of all supplements or medical foods you are taking regularly. Make a list and share it with everyone even if you think they don't understand or support you. This is very important.

SOME IMPORTANT REMINDERS

1. Do not take any additional antioxidants for one day before and at least two days after any treatment to optimize treatment. Antioxidants may interfere with the clearance of some chemotherapy agents
2. Eat small amounts of food every few hours rather than big meals. You may find your appetite is best in the morning; this is a good time to eat a healthy breakfast. Don't go for longer than eight hours overnight without something with calories as this is when your body needs energy the most. Try sipping papaya or apricot nectar or pineapple juice if you wake up as these are easy to digest.
3. Drink plenty of fluids; use water, clear soups and juices in preference to caffeinated beverages.
4. Imagine your digestion as that of a young child. Eat only small quantities at a time of easy to digest foods. Small jars of weaning baby food may be helpful as ready-to-eat supplemental snack meals. Protein smoothies are useful to sip on. Try garnishing them with fresh fruit to make them more appealing.
5. Microwave or moist cook fruits and vegetables to improve their digestibility.
6. If fruit upsets your stomach, use juice instead. You can also dilute it with water.
7. Experiment with different foods in small amounts. Everyone's digestion is unique. Some people find spicy foods helpful while others do not.

Remember we are all different. There is no right or wrong way to eat; we have different cultures, different personal histories with food as well as different tastes. Staying healthy and strong is what is important.

HERBS AND SURGERY WARNINGS

The American Medical Association recently issued the following warnings about herbs that should be discontinued prior to surgery:

Herb	Discontinue Period Prior to Surgery

Ephedra	At least 24 hours before surgery
Garlic	At least 7 days before surgery
Ginkgo	At least 36 hours before surgery
Ginseng	At least 7 days before surgery
Kava	At least 24 hours before surgery
St. John's Wort	At least 5 days before surgery
Valerian	Taper off several weeks before surgery. Suddenly stopping can cause withdrawal problems.

Source:
Use of Herbal Medications before Surgery. Betz et al. JAMA.2001; 286: 2542-2544.

TELL YOUR MEDICAL TEAM ABOUT ANY SUPPLEMENTS YOU ARE TAKING.

FOODS FOR OPTIMAL HEALTH

Every day you consume some 23,000 different chemicals. Most of these chemicals need to be metabolized before excretion and in order to protect from potential toxicity or damage we need to eat foods regularly that support this complex system of enzymes. Foods rich in the 3 A's (Antioxidants, Anti-carcinogens and Anti-inflammatories) may be helpful in promoting healthy liver function and support of immune health. They include the following:

Acorn squash
Asparagus
Avocado
Bitter melon
Blackberries
Black currants
Blueberries
Cantaloupe
Cruciferous vegetable family
Garlic
Grapes
Green tea
Orange (especially the zest from the rind)
Pomegranates
Potatoes
Parsley
Raspberries
Spinach
Strawberries
Tomatoes
Turmeric
Walnuts
Zucchini

Suggested Supplements

Multivitamin and mineral	One daily with food
Alpha Lipoic Acid	60 milligrams daily
Coenzyme Q10	120 milligrams daily
Selenium	200 micrograms daily
Vitamin D	400 IU (up to 2,000 IU per day)
Vitamin E (as mixed tocopherols)	200 IU daily

During treatment (optional and only with oncologist approval)

Astragalus root	1 capsule (Solgar)
Milk thistle (Silymarin)	80 milligrams (Solgar)
Mushroom extract	as directed, e.g. Andrew Weil's Origins

SUGGESTIONS FOR HANDLING TREATMENT SIDE EFFECTS

Eating well is vital to give you that extra edge as you participate in your own recovery. Choose healthy foods to empower yourself for this important time in your life. Each time you choose a fruit, vegetable or protein rich food you are giving your body what it needs to fight the cancer. Improved nutrition can also help you to withstand the side effects of chemotherapy, radiation and surgery. Some treatments may make eating difficult or distasteful but there are many valuable medications available to minimize side effects. Remember to ask ahead so you can prevent rather than treat nausea, diarrhea and constipation.

Here are some specific nutrition suggestions to help you with some of the most common treatment-related problems. Even if some of these ideas appear to be in conflict with the basic high fiber/low saturated animal fat concepts you are familiar with, maintaining a reasonably constant body weight is your overriding priority at this time. Choose fats or oils that contain more of the beneficial fatty acids to boost calories as well as support your immunity. Examples include olives (and olive oil), avocados, nuts (almonds, walnuts and Brazil nuts are particularly good - nut butters are valuable ways of consuming them) and seeds (sunflower or pumpkin).

Suggestions for chewing and swallowing difficulties:

1. Eat foods prepared with moist heat such as soups, stews, casseroles or pasta.
2. Add gravy, sauces, butter, mayonnaise or salad dressings to make food easier to swallow.
3. Avoid highly seasoned, spicy, tart or acidic foods such as tomatoes.
4. Avoid alcohol and smoking.
5. Cold foods may be soothing if there are sores in the mouth. Use a straw. Ice chips or popsicles may be helpful.
6. Keep your caloric intake high by using protein smoothies and meal replacement drinks, e.g. Resource Plus®, Prosure® or Resurgex®
7. If you have trouble swallowing soups, try using a cup or glass instead of a spoon.
8. Try carbonated drinks as they may be easier to swallow. Carbonation often helps with nausea by releasing upper gas. Try ginger ale as ginger is also good for preventing nausea.

Suggestions for dealing with diarrhea:

1. Choose oatmeal, white rice and other refined grain products.
2. Chicken noodle soup is an old standby; home made is best.

3. Avoid eating raw fruits and vegetables except bananas. Peel all vegetables before cooking and remove skins and seeds. Avoid nuts and popcorn.
4. Avoid high fiber foods that contain a great deal of roughage; for instance wheat bran, wheat germ or whole wheat. Iceberg lettuce, onions, garlic, cucumber and celery may also cause intestinal distress.
5. Eat cooked apples, apple sauce or apple puree. These are binding.
6. Don't drink more than 1 cup of fluid with your meals, but drink plenty of water in between.
7. Eat frequent, small meals rather than three large ones.
8. Food and liquids should be warm or at room temperature, rather than very hot or ice cold.
9. If the diarrhea is severe, restrict your diet to clear liquids such as broth, lemon barley water, flat ginger ale, tea or sports types of drinks (Gatorade or Powerade) for one day. If it persists for more than one day, call your physician.

Suggestions for dealing with constipation:

1. Drink plenty of fluids. At least 1 liter of water daily.
2. Eat prunes, apricots, peaches, cherries or other pitted fruit
3. Drink prune juice.
4. Use syrup of figs as a gentle laxative.
5. Eat rhubarb (only the red parts, stewed).
6. Add wheat bran or wheat germ to breakfast cereals.
7. Exercise, stretching and all types of movements help stimulate circulation which may ease constipation. Avoid sitting for long periods.
8. Maintain a regular morning schedule allowing plenty of time.
9. Try a hot drink and then relax. Avoid straining.

Suggestions for dealing with nausea and/or vomiting:

1. Eat and drink slowly.
2. Eat small, frequent meals, chewed well.
3. Try ginger ale or crystallized ginger.
4. Avoid greasy, fatty and fried foods.
5. Rest after meals.
6. For early morning or pre-meal nausea, try a cracker or dry toast.
7. Make up for lost calories when you feel more comfortable.
8. Avoid cooking odors by microwaving. Use a fan in the kitchen.
9. Try crushed ice types of drinks.

Suggestions for loss of appetite:

1. If you aren't hungry at dinner time, make breakfast or lunch your main meal. Similarly, if you aren't hungry first thing in the morning, eat more later.
2. Eat more frequently, but smaller amounts of food.
3. Keep snacks readily available, e.g. in your purse or in the car.
4. Always make food look attractive with garnishes or with place settings.
5. Experiment with tastes - you may find things you didn't like before, you like now.
6. Cold or room temperature foods may be more appealing.
7. A glass of wine or beer may increase your appetite (check with your doctor first in case alcohol doesn't mix with your medication).
8. Increase the caloric intake of the foods that you do eat with a small amount of "light" (less strongly flavored, not fewer calories) olive oil.

9. Try a protein smoothie or one of the commercially prepared meal replacement drinks such as Prosure®, Ensure® or Boost®. Whey protein powder is easy to digest and nutritious. Please visit my website at www.cancernutrition.com for more suggestions.

SUGGESTIONS FOR EATING TO PROVIDE MAXIMUM IMMUNITY

By making wise eating choices, you may be able to fortify your natural defenses and handle treatments with ease. Remember to take extra care with personal hygiene such as having regular manicures and pedicures along with taking care to wash your hands frequently as your immune system may be compromised due to treatment. Listen to your body's needs for rest and sleep. You will benefit from being in natural surroundings and by keeping the company of those who support rather than drain you of energy. Stay away from negative people and negative news that you can't do anything about - you need all the strength for yourself right now.

As each person's nutritional needs are very individual, I suggest that you see a nutritionist or Registered Dietitian (RD) at this time to assist you in making healthy food choices. Make a weekly food and exercise diary and place it on the refrigerator. This way you can monitor your changes in a way that is valuable for you, your family and your health care team.

The following essential nutrients maintain healthy immunity:

Nutrient	Food Source
Vitamin A	Fish liver oils, liver
Lycopene and carotenes	Red, orange, yellow and dark green vegetables including watermelon, pink grapefruit, cantaloupe, apricots and spinach
Vitamin B1 (Thiamin)	Whole grains, fortified breakfast cereals
Vitamin B2 (Riboflavin)	Whole and enriched cereals and breads, lean meat, milk, eggs and organic liver
Vitamin B3 (Niacin)	Whole grains, eggs, liver
Vitamin B6 (Pyridoxine)	Whole grains, lean meat, eggs, organic liver
Folic acid	Whole grains, leafy vegetables, meat
Pantothenic acid	Brewer's yeast, beans, salmon
Vitamin C	Citrus fruits, kiwi, strawberries, peppers
Vitamin D	Oily fish (salmon, sardines), fortified dairy products
Vitamin E	Egg yolk, liver, wheat germ, nuts and seeds
Iron	Liver, egg yolk, green peas, asparagus
Magnesium	Leafy vegetables, nuts, seafood
Manganese	Bananas, bran, pineapple, nuts
Potassium	Citrus fruit, mushrooms
Selenium	Garlic, legumes, fish, asparagus
Sulfur	Garlic, avocado, lean meat
Zinc	Oysters, liver, sunflower seeds
Phytochemicals	Dark pigmented herbs, berries
Antioxidants	Blueberries, cocoa, red grapes, kiwi, culinary herbs
Protein	Eggs, lean meat, poultry, fish, shellfish

SUGAR

Does sugar feed cancer? This question is the most common one I receive on my website. The answer is not a simple one as we are all different and cancer itself is not one disease but a multitude of different genetic mutations. If you have a glucose sensitive metabolism or if your particular cancer has resulted in changes in glucose sensitivity then sugar may be feeding your cancer and we recommend that you reduce your intake to less than 30 grams per day or not exceeding 14 grams per meal or per drink. This won't harm anyone but is particularly important for some people. Most cancer cells develop the capacity to use energy from glucose (one of the two components of table sugar or sucrose) without needing oxygen. This means that the cells are able to survive when most other cells cannot. We can't live without glucose or oxygen however, as we need both for all of our healthy cells. Glucose is the preferred fuel for the brain and liver.

INFLAMMATORY PROCESSES AND CANCER

Inflammation is thought to play a critical role in cancer processes. Anti-inflammatory foods are important for everyone and are especially important for those dealing with cancer. Anti-inflammatory foods fight inflammatory processes. Omega-3 oils are important anti-inflammatory foods and are found in blue-green algae and spirulina. Ocean fish consume these tiny plant-like substances and concentrate them and thus the fish then become excellent sources of omega-3 oils. Krill oil is also an excellent source of omega-3 fatty acids. Salmon, herrings and sardines are some of the richest sources of these important oils that enhance anti-inflammatory processes in the body. Omega-3 oils are important in all nervous system functions. A panel of nutritionists and scientists at the National Institutes of Health recently recommended that a ratio of omega-6 (thought to be pro-inflammatory) to omega-3 (anti-inflammatory) oils should ideally be 4. The usual dietary intake in the United States is currently about 10-20:1 omega-6: omega-3. The best way to adjust the ratio is to cut down on omega-6 and include more omega-3 rich foods such as salmon, pine nuts and walnuts. You may also wish to include a supplement of EPA and DHA (the principle omega-3 oils). Personally, I like spirulina. Omega-3 oils are found in oily fish, nuts such as walnuts, macadamia, pecans and certain seeds and vegetables. GLA (Gamma linoleic acid) is an important oil found in flaxseed. Evening primrose, black currant seed and borage are other supplemental sources. GLA is good for regulating hormone and prostaglandins (short acting local hormones). GLA may be taken as a supplement.

Anti-inflammatory processes are favored when you balance your sources of oils and fats:

Choose oily fish, nuts and seeds often
Watch your intake of cheese, butter and bacon
Use cold pressed extra virgin olive oil (EVO) in salad dressings
Sprinkle pine nuts on salads
Choose avocado often

Other sources of Anti-inflammatory nutrients

Many fruits and vegetables are rich in anti-inflammatory aspirin like substances also called COX-inhibitors. Examples include apricots, broccoli, turmeric, raspberries, loganberries, pineapple, curry, rosemary, thyme and tarragon. Choose foods often that have properties of **the 3 A's** - anticarcinogenic (against cancer), anti-oxidant and anti-inflammatory

ANTICARCINOGENS ANTIOXIDANTS ANTI INFLAMMATORIES

DIGESTIVE ENZYMES

What are digestive enzymes?

Digestive enzymes are proteins that assist in the digestion of food. They are also thought to assist in maintaining health at the cellular level and are often recommended for cancer patients during and after treatment.

Proteases help break down proteins
Amylases help break down carbohydrates
Lipases help break down fats and oils

Do I need to take an enzyme supplement?

Some people benefit from taking supplemental digestive enzymes especially during chemotherapy or after radiation to the digestive tract region. Digestive enzymes can reduce abdominal discomfort and gas. Wobenzyme-N is a good example of a high quality digestive enzyme supplement containing bromelain (from pineapple) and papain (from papaya).

Which foods contain digestive enzymes?

Pineapple, papaya and guava are good sources of proteases. Noni and mangosteen juices may also be valuable.

Are these supplements safe to take?

Yes, these are safe supplements and may enhance white cell activity which is often helpful during chemotherapy.

IF SOMEONE YOU LOVE HAS CANCER

Learning that someone you love has cancer may be one of the most frightening moments of your life. This is often because of the things we have heard or read that make it sound like a death sentence. However, this simply isn't true. Today there are more than 10 million cancer survivors in America and for most people who are diagnosed with cancer, it will not be the reason for their death. Heart disease is the leading cause of death for the age group that is most affected by cancer. One of the most important things you can do for yourself and for your loved one is to find out exactly what the facts are about their diagnosis. The American Cancer Society is the most respected and trusted source of cancer information and they can be reached 24 hours a day (toll free) at 1-800-4CANCER or on their website www.cancer.org I encourage you to gather relevant paperwork such as copies of biopsy and blood test results and keep them in a folder. Write down questions to ask the medical professionals and write down the answers received. Many people find that keeping records lowers their anxiety level and gives them a feeling of control.

Typical questions might be:

What is my diagnosis? What stage is my cancer at?
How aggressive is the cancer?
How long will I receive treatment for?
How will I feel after my treatments?
Is there anything I should avoid?
Can I continue to exercise?
Are there foods I should avoid?
Is the treatment likely to make me feel nauseated?
Is the treatment likely to give me diarrhea/constipation?
Are there over the counter medications I should have on hand?

How will I know how I am progressing?
How often will I have scans/blood tests?
Is there a clinical trial I am eligible for?

SADNESS, DEPRESSION AND OTHER FACTORS AFFECTING APPETITE

Stress can take a toll on your digestion so I would recommend choosing foods that you enjoy and that are easy to assimilate. Soups, cooked starches such as pasta, baked potato, rice and plain baked goods are examples of easily digested foods. You may wish to choose a favorite food that reminds you of happier times. Comfort foods are just that and when eaten in small quantities on special occasions they warm the heart. If you or a loved one are feeling sad ask these few questions:

1) Am I eating breakfast regularly?
2) Am I taking my supplements and medications regularly (if applicable)?
3) Am I sleeping at least seven hours a night?
4) Am I spending time outside every day?
5) Have I spoken to at least one friend or family member in the past twenty four hours?
6) Am I skipping meals more often?
7) Is my refrigerator almost empty?
8) Am I overeating (or undereating)?
9) Am I eating empty calories more often?
10) Am I avoiding shopping for food?

If you answered NO to questions 1-5 and/or YES to questions 6-10, then you may benefit from visiting a health professional.

SAMPLE FOOD CHOICES

Breakfast choices

Whole grain type of dry cereal
Eggs (poached, scrambled, boiled or as an omelet)
Oatmeal or other hot cereal
Whole grain bread, toast or bagel

Snack

Fresh fruit
Small protein smoothie (4-6 fluid ounces)
Yogurt

Lunch

Ginger-sesame salmon
Brown rice
Asparagus spears topped with slivered almonds
OR
Chicken breast and walnuts
Garlic mashed potatoes
Red cabbage
OR
Bean, noodle and nut deep dish
Salad of leafy, young dark greens topped with
Balsamic vinegar and extra virgin olive oil salad dressing

OR
Vegetable curry
Brown rice
Fruit chutney
OR
Lentil and pecan deep dish
Grated carrots, beets and radish salad
Olive oil and rice vinegar salad dressing
OR
White fish with fresh ginger and lemon
Brown rice
Spinach with olive oil and garlic
OR
Frittata with spinach
Tomato and Maui onion salad
Extra virgin olive oil and pine nuts

Snack

Small handful of dried apricots and almonds
Ginger snap cookie and milk

Dinner

Pasta primavera
Asparagus tips garnish
Small side salad
OR
Stir-fry vegetables on bed of brown rice
OR
Tasty rice and tofu
Spinach salad with slivered almonds
Olive oil and balsamic vinegar dressing
OR
Halibut with broccoli and almonds
Brown rice
Sliced buffalo tomatoes
OR
Sea bass with apples
Mashed potatoes
Brussels sprouts and chestnuts
Cherry tomatoes
OR
Teriyaki salmon
Fingerling potatoes
Broccolini (steamed)
Garlic and parsley butter topping
OR
Risotto

Salad of mixed dark leafy greens
Olive oil and balsamic vinegar dressing

Desserts and comfort foods

Fruit Brown Betty
Egg custard
Ice cream (made with high quality ingredients)

By the bedside

Apricot or guava nectar
Graham crackers

When selecting your or a loved one's menu plans remember that taste buds may be affected by the treatment. Adjust seasonings accordingly and avoid strong flavors that may irritate mouth and gums. Create an eating environment that is as stress free as possible; add flowers to your table or tray setting and avoid challenging conversations or other upsetting distractions. Many people enjoy eating in restaurants because they don't have to choose what to eat hours ahead, someone else cleans up and the environment is usually quiet and supportive. Some people enjoy a glass of wine with their evening meal. It is a good idea to eat the most in the morning or at midday. Our bodies have a natural circadian rhythm that encourages us to eat earlier in the day so we can move around and digest best. Eating a lot in the evening isn't recommended as it may interfere with restful sleep.

SOME DIET SUGGESTIONS

To increase calories

Add avocado to salads or sandwiches. Slice in half and squeeze fresh lemon or lime juice, twisting the rind to extract essential oils such as limonene which are important at inducing apoptosis (programmed cell death).
Add olive or hazelnut oil to vegetables
Be generous with salad dressings

To increase protein

Add protein powder to fruit juices and smoothies
Include cottage cheese often
Add hard boiled eggs and egg whites to salads
Add skim dry milk powder to recipes

To increase cancer fighting phytonutrients or botanical factors

Choose asparagus often
Drink pomegranate juice (1-2 fluid ounces)
Choose curry, cook with turmeric and cumin
Choose blueberries, raspberries and cranberries often
Choose rhubarb

To increase iron

Choose peas
Choose eggs (yolk is rich in iron)
Choose asparagus
Choose organic lamb or chicken liver

To increase magnesium

Choose dark green leafy vegetables
Choose nuts and nut butters

To increase potassium

Choose to squeeze the juice and add zest of fresh lemon or lime in your water
Choose mushrooms
Choose bananas

Each time you select a food with additional benefits you are making a positive health move. This is empowering and your body will thank you.

SUGGESTED ITEMS TO HAVE ON HAND

You may wish to have some items on hand for times when you don't feel like shopping. These are some things to consider: Milk (you can purchase shelf stable cartons of low fat flavored types), fruit yogurt, chicken breast, almond cookies, soup ingredients (or a can of healthy low sodium minestrone), canned beans, spaghetti, dried fruit, dark chocolate with almonds.

You may wish to vary your menus. Try writing them out and posting them in your kitchen. This helps you feel more secure and cared for. If you are caring for a loved one, menu planning shows your thoughtfulness.

There are several other non nutritional items that may be helpful such as gentle laxatives or stool softeners, anti-diarrhea remedies, soothing types of mouthwash (ask your nursing staff for suitable combinations), antihistamines and sleep aids.

Have some movies on hand that make you laugh, those that are sentimental and maybe even some dramas so you can lift your mood with an entertainment distraction. You may also wish to have some flowering plants and herbs placed around your home. Choose uplifting and enriching decorative items so your home environment is healing. Whenever possible go outside and enjoy the fresh air and beauty of nature.

MY DAILY FOOD GUIDE

Food I choose to eat	Liquids	How I feel	Notes

Summary of My Day

Appetite: Fluids: Other information:

Make as many copies of this page as you need and post on the refrigerator for your health team members to help assist you in providing the care you need.

HELPFUL RECIPES

If your mouth is sore:

Babaghanoush 24
Chicken and Okra Gumbo 26
Green Pea Soup 28
Root Vegetable Soup 31
Brown Rice Pilaf (cook well) 34
Risotto 39
Spaghetti with Artichoke Hearts 40
Tasty Rice and Tofu 41
Creamy Dijon Sole 44
Garlic Mashed Potatoes 53
Angel Food Cake 58
Key Lime Pie 61
Apple Pie Smoothie 65
Banana Fruit Smoothie 66
Black Forest Smoothie 66
Cappuccino Smoothie 66
Extra Chocolatey Smoothie 67
Passionate Papaya Smoothie 68
Peach Milk Smoothie 69
Soda Fountain Shake 70
Vanilla Shake 71

If you are constipated:

Bean Dip 24
Guacamole 26
Chicken Soup 27
Gazpacho 27
Green Pea Soup 28
Immuno-Soup 29
Minestrone 30
Phytomineral Soup 30
Root Vegetable 31
Adzuki Beans and Rice 32
Baked Beans 33
Bean, Noodle and Nut Casserole 33
Blackeyed Peas 34
Flageolets 35
Lentil and Pecan Casserole 35
Lentil Patties 36
Mexican Bean Pie 36
Navy Bean Stew 37
Pasta Primavera 38

Quinoa-Nut Vegetable Pilaf 39
Spaghetti with Artichoke Hearts 40
Southern Style Beans and Rice 40
Tasty Rice and Tofu 41
Broiled Orange Roughy 43
Monkfish, Mushrooms and Lentils 45
Sea Bass with Apples 46
White Fish with Ginger and Lemon 48
Brussels Sprouts and Chestnuts 51
Eggplant Parmesan 51
French Peas 52
Spinach, Brown Rice and Tofu 55
Sweet and Sour Vegetables 56
Vegetable Curry 56
Vegetarian Stew 57
Apricot and Strawberry Cake 59
Ginger Cookies 60
Fresh Fruit Salad 63
Pears in Red Wine 64
Apple Pie Smoothie 65
Banana Fruit Smoothie 66
Black Forest Smoothie 66
Extra Chocolatey Smoothie 67
Passionate Papaya Smoothie 68
Prune Smoothie 69
Raspberry RazMaTaz 69
Strawberry Daiquiri 71
Strawberry Sensation 71

If you have diarrhea:
Miso soup 30
Cinnamon Applesauce 62

If your blood count is low:
Chicken Liver Pâté 25

APPETIZERS

Babaghanoush

- 2 medium eggplants
- 1 tablespoon lemon juice
- 1 tablespoon tahini
- 2 tablespoons fresh parsley, chopped
- 1 pinch cumin powder (optional)
- 1 ½ tablespoons nonfat yogurt
- 1 clove garlic, crushed

Bake the eggplant in a medium oven at 350 degrees until cooked through (about 20 minutes). Remove the skin and place in a blender. Add the tahini, yogurt, garlic, lemon juice and cumin powder. Blend to desired consistency. Season to taste and chill before serving. Garnish with chopped parsley.

Note: Good source of Folic acid

Serves 4

Prep Time: 0:25

Calories 90	Carbohydrate 16g	Cholesterol 0mg
Protein 4g	Fat 2g	Dietary Fiber 3g
	% Calories from fat 22%	

Bean Dip

- ½ cup beans, soaked overnight
- ½ tablespoon extra virgin olive oil
- 2 tablespoons salsa
- 1 tablespoon fresh chives, chopped
- ¼ teaspoon salt
- ¼ teaspoon black pepper

Rinse and drain the beans (any type is good). Boil for 20 minutes or until tender. If using canned beans, drain. Transfer to a blender and blend until smooth. Add the salsa, oil, salt and black pepper and continue to blend. Place in a serving bowl and chill. Serve with blue corn chips as an appetizer.

Notes: Excellent source of Folic acid. Good source of Vitamin B1. You can use the recipe for Salsa or purchase ready mixed salsa. Canned beans may also be used.

Serves: 5

Prep Time: 0:30

Calories: 106	Carbohydrate 16g	Cholesterol 0mg
Protein 6g	Fat 2g	Dietary Fiber 6g
	% Calories from fat 19%	

Bruschetta

- 4 slices Italian bread
- 2 garlic cloves
- ½ tablespoon olive oil
- 4 plum tomatoes, sliced
- 2 tablespoons fresh basil, chopped
- ½ teaspoon black pepper, fresh ground

Use a broiler to toast the bread on both sides. Rub the upper surfaces with garlic and sprinkle with olive oil.

Top with slices of tomato and sprinkle with fresh basil and black pepper. Serve immediately while the toast is still warm.

Notes: Excellent source of Vitamin C and lycopene. Good source of Vitamin A, B1, B2, Folate and Niacin.

Serves: 4
Prep Time: 0:15

Calories 123	Carbohydrate 21g	Cholesterol 0mg
Protein 4g	Fat 3g	Dietary Fiber 2g
	% Calories from fat 22%	

Chicken Liver Pâté

- ¾ pound chicken livers
- ½ medium Spanish onion
- 1 stalk celery, finely chopped
- ¼ green bell pepper, finely chopped
- 2 egg whites, hard boiled
- ¼ teaspoon salt
- ½ teaspoon black pepper
- 1 teaspoon olive oil

In a non stick skillet sprayed with olive oil, gently sauté the chicken livers for 2-3 minutes until firm but not completely cooked through. Place the livers and hard boiled egg whites together in a blender and blend until smooth. Add the celery and green bell pepper and combine by hand with the seasonings. Place in a pâté dish or small soufflé dish and chill in the refrigerator. A thin layer of clarified butter on top will keep the pâté fresh for a few days in the refrigerator. Serve garnished with a little chopped parsley and with triangles of thinly sliced toast.

Notes: Excellent source of Vitamin C, A, B6, B12, B2, Folate, Niacin and Iron. Good source of Zinc.
If you like pâté, this is a lower fat, lower cholesterol version that still retains good flavor. Liver pâté is a nutritious appetizer.

Serves: 6
Prep Time: 0:05
Stand Time: 0:30

Calories 90	Carbohydrate 4 g	Cholesterol 249 mg
Protein 12 g	Fat 3g	Dietary Fiber 0g.
	% Calories from fat 30%	

Curry Dip

- ½ cup plain low fat yogurt
- 2 teaspoons curry powder
- 1 teaspoon fresh lemon juice
- 2 drops Tabasco sauce
- ¼ teaspoon black pepper
- 1 teaspoon sugar

Combine the ingredients together and place in a serving dish. Garnish with cayenne or paprika. Serve with crackers and fresh vegetables.

Note: Good source of Vitamin C.

Serves: 4
Prep Time: 0:05

Calories 20	Carbohydrate 3g	Cholesterol 1mg
Protein 1g	Fat 2g	Dietary Fiber 0g
	% Calories from fat 18%	

Guacamole

- 2 avocados
- ¼ cup fresh lemon juice
- 1 clove garlic, crushed
- 6 tomatoes, peeled and chopped
- 1 medium onion, chopped
- 1 green bell pepper, peeled and chopped
- 1 tablespoon fresh cilantro, finely chopped
- ½ teaspoon salt
- ¼ teaspoon black pepper

Peel, remove the pit and mash the avocado. Add the lemon juice, garlic, tomatoes, onion and pepper. Stir in the cilantro. Replace the avocado pit to keep the guacamole from turning brown. Serve with corn chips.

Notes: Excellent source of Vitamin C, A, B6, Folate. Good source of Vitamin B1, B2, Niacin and Iron. Eat sparingly as this is a high-fat food. Fat content is of good fatty acid profile and this dish is a good source of antioxidants and glutathione which is supportive to liver health.

Serves: 4
Prep Time: 0:10

Calories 214	Carbohydrate 19g	Cholesterol 0mg
Protein 4g	Fat 16g	Dietary Fiber 5g
	% Calories from fat 60%	

SOUPS

Chicken and Okra Gumbo

- 2 chicken breast halves, skinless
- 2 tablespoons olive oil
- 2 cups chopped okra
- 1 medium chopped onion
- 2 sticks chopped celery
- 1 medium chopped green bell pepper
- 4 garlic cloves, crushed
- 1 tablespoon Worcestershire sauce
- ½ teaspoon Creole seasoning
- ½ cup cooked rice
- 3 quarts water

Garnish

- 1 can (15 ounces tomatoes)
- 1 tablespoon chopped scallions
- ¼ teaspoon filé (optional)

Heat half of the oil in a heavy-bottomed casserole dish. Dust the chicken with flour and brown for 4-6 minutes on each side. Remove and set aside in a warm place. Add the rest of the oil and sauté the okra for 10 minutes stirring constantly. Add the onion, celery, bell pepper and garlic and continue to cook for 1-2 minutes. Add the chicken, tomatoes, Worcestershire sauce, seasonings and water and bring to a boil. Reduce the heat, cover the pan and simmer for 2 hours or until the chicken is tender. Skim excess fat and serve with rice in soup bowls. Garnish with chopped scallions and a sprinkling of filé, if available.

Notes: Excellent source of Vitamin C, B6 and Folate Good source of Vitamin A, B1 and Niacin.
Serving Size: 6
Prep Time: 0:20
Cooking Time: 2:00 hours

Calories 109
Protein 9g
Carbohydrate 13g
Fat 3g
% Calories from fat 24%
Cholesterol 17mg
Dietary Fiber 2g

Chicken Soup

3 pounds chicken, skinless light meat cut in pieces
4 quarts water
2 bay leaves
½ teaspoon pepper
1 teaspoon paprika
3 cloves crushed garlic
3 medium sliced carrots
3 stalks chopped celery
1 medium chopped onion
2 sliced leeks
2 sprigs parsley
½ tablespoon olive oil

Heat the oil in a large, heavy based pan. Sauté the onions and garlic for 3-4 minutes. Add the water, paprika, salt, pepper and bay leaves. Bring to a boil, cover and simmer for 2 hours. Remove from the heat, cut the chicken into small pieces and remove the bones. Return the chicken to the pan and add the carrots, celery and parsley. Simmer for another hour. Serve hot.

Notes: Excellent source of Vitamin C, A, B6, B12, B2, Niacin, Calcium, Iron and Zinc. Good source of Vitamin B1 and Folate.
Serving Size: 4
Prep Time: 0:10
Cooking Time: 3:00 hours

Calories 332
Protein 48g
Carbohydrate 25g
Fat 6g
% Calories from fat 16%
Cholesterol 99mg
Dietary Fiber 6g

Gazpacho

1 clove crushed garlic
6 cups chopped tomatoes
1 medium chopped onion
½ cup chopped green pepper
½ cup chopped cucumber
¼ cup fine ground breadcrumbs
2 cups tomato juice
½ teaspoon cumin
½ teaspoon ground black pepper
½ teaspoon salt
1 tablespoon extra virgin olive oil
¼ cup fresh lemon juice

Blend the tomatoes, garlic, onion and green pepper in a blender. Add the cucumber and strain into a serving bowl containing the breadcrumbs. Mix well and chill for 30 minutes in the refrigerator. Before serving, blend the olive oil, lemon juice, salt, pepper, cumin and tomato juice. Stir into the mixture and serve garnished with small dishes of diced tomatoes, cucumber and green pepper.

Notes: Excellent source of Vitamin A, C, B6 and Folate. Good source of Calcium.
Serving Size: 6
Prep Time: 0:10
Stand Time: 0:30

Calories 112	Carbohydrate 20g	Cholesterol 0mg
Protein 4g	Fat 3g	Dietary Fiber 4g
	% Calories from fat 23%	

Green Pea Soup

- ½ tablespoon olive oil
- 2 medium chopped onions
- 2 stalks chopped celery
- 1½ cups split peas
- 4 cups water
- 1 teaspoon oregano
- 1 teaspoon black pepper
- ½ teaspoon salt
- ½ teaspoon dry mustard

Soak the split peas overnight and drain the water. Heat the oil in a saucepan and sauté the onions and celery for 3-4 minutes. Add the celery and cook for another 2 minutes. Add the water and peas and bring to a boil. Cover and simmer for 20 minutes or until the peas become mushy. Place in a blender or food processor with a metal blade to blend. Add oregano and adjust seasoning. Serve hot with croutons.

Notes: Excellent source of Vitamin B1 and Folate. Good source of Vitamin B6, Iron and Zinc.
Serving Size: 6
Prep Time: 0:30 (overnight for soaking of split peas)

Calories 192	Carbohydrate 33	Cholesterol 0g
Protein 13g	Fat 2g	Dietary Fiber 14g
	% Calories from fat 8%	

Immuno-Soup

- 1 cup beans (red kidney, pinto, etc.), soaked overnight or canned
- 2 whole carrots, sliced thin
- 1 whole beet, sliced
- 1 whole potato, diced
- 1 head celery, chopped
- 1 bunch parsley, chopped
- ½ pounds sliced green beans
- 4 whole zucchini, sliced thin
- 1 whole rutabaga or parsnip, chopped
- 1 whole turnip, chopped
- 2 cloves crushed garlic
- ½ bell pepper, chopped
- ½ teaspoon oregano
- ½ teaspoon marjoram
- ½ teaspoon rosemary

1 bunch scallions, sliced	½ teaspoon sage
1 pound spinach, chopped	1 teaspoon thyme
½ head cauliflower, broken in pieces	

Soak beans overnight and discard water. Wash and prepare the vegetables. Place the root vegetables (carrots, potatoes, turnip, parsnip or rutabaga) into a large pot with the beans. Half fill the pot with water and bring to a boil. Cover and simmer for 10 minutes. Add all of the other ingredients and season to taste. Return to a boil and cook uncovered for 1-2 minutes more. Cover and simmer for another 30 minutes. Adjust seasoning and serve hot or cold.

This soup improves with age. Split into to 1-2 cup-sized servings and freeze for a quick and healthy meal. You can add grated cheese to the surface of a bowl and melt it under a hot grill. For variety include brown rice, barley, noodles or corn. Tamari, soy sauce or Bragg's liquid aminos also add flavor.

Notes: Excellent source of Vitamin C, A, B6, B1, B2, Folate, Calcium and Iron. Good source of Niacin and Zinc. Serving Idea: Serve with hot crusty bread.

Serving Size: 8
Prep Time: 0:45

Calories 179	Carbohydrate 35g	Cholesterol 0mg
Protein 12g	Fat 1g	Dietary Fiber 13g
	% Calories from fat 5%	

Minestrone

1 cup white beans, soaked	½ cup frozen green peas
½ tablespoon olive oil	½ cup frozen chopped green beans
1 medium chopped onion	½ teaspoon rosemary
2 cloves crushed garlic	½ teaspoon thyme
2 stalks chopped celery	½ teaspoon oregano
3 medium diced carrots	½ teaspoon marjoram
1 diced green bell pepper	½ cup cooked pasta shells
8 cups water	1 teaspoon salt
	½ teaspoon black pepper

Rinse the beans and boil for 20 minutes. Heat the oil in a non-stick skillet and sauté the onion and garlic for 3-4 minutes. Add the celery, carrots and green pepper and continue to cook for 1-2 minutes. Add the water, salt and pepper and bring to a boil, cover and simmer for 15 minutes. Add the pasta shells, green beans and peas and continue to cook for 10 minutes. Serve hot.

Notes: Excellent source of Vitamin C, A, B1, Folate and Iron. Good source of Vitamin B6, Calcium and Zinc.

Serving Size: 6
Prep Time: 1:00

Calories 192	Carbohydrate 35g	Cholesterol 0mg

Protein 11g	Fat 1g	Dietary Fiber 8g
	% Calories from fat 7%	

Miso Soup

2 ounces inaka miso (country style)
5 ounces silken bean curd diced
3 cups dashi stock

Put dashi stock into a pan. Add miso and stir until dissolved. Add bean curd and heat. Do not allow to boil. Serve garnished with finely sliced green onions.

**dashi stock
2.5 x 1.5 inches dried kelp
50 grams dried bonito flakes
7 cups water

Wipe the kelp with a damp cloth. Cover with water and heat. Just before the water boils remove the kelp and discard. Sprinkle bonito flakes and strain as the flakes begin to sink.

Notes: Good source of Vitamin B12
Serving Size: 4
Prep Time: 0:15

Calories 58	Carbohydrates 5g	Cholesterol 3mg
Protein 6g	Fat 2g	Dietary Fiber 1g
	% Calories from fat 31%	

Phytomineral Soup

1 medium chopped onion
2 sticks chopped celery
4 cloves crushed garlic
1 teaspoon curry powder
2 medium sliced carrots
½ cup corn
1 15 ounce can tomatoes
1 packet vegetable bouillon cubes
1 cup frozen peas
½ cup firm tofu
2 cups spinach leaves, chopped
½ cup chopped parsley
1 teaspoon thyme
½ teaspoon rosemary
1 tablespoon olive oil
5 cups water
a pinch salt
¼ teaspoon black pepper

Heat the oil in a large non-stick skillet. Sauté the onions and garlic for 3-5 minutes. Add the celery and carrots and sauté for a further 2 minutes. Add the corn, tomatoes, parsley, thyme, rosemary and sage. Dissolve the packet of vegetable broth in a cup of boiling water. Add to the pan with 4 more cups of water. Bring to a boil, cover and reduce the heat. Simmer for 20 minutes. Add the peas, tofu and spinach. Season to taste and simmer for 5 more minutes.

Notes: Excellent source of Vitamin C, A, B6, Folate and Iron. Good source of Vitamin B1, B2, Niacin, Calcium and Zinc.
Serving Size: 6

Prep Time: 0:30

Calories 153	Carbohydrate 23g	Cholesterol 0mg
Protein 7g	Fat 4g	Dietary Fiber 4g
	% Calories from fat 24%	

Rice and Celery Soup

- 6 sticks celery, finely chopped
- 1 cup rice
- 2 chicken bouillon cubes
- 6 cups water
- ½ medium chopped onion
- 1 can (15 ounces) tomatoes
- 1 tablespoon extra virgin olive oil
- ½ teaspoon salt
- ½ cup fresh parsley, finely chopped
- ½ teaspoon black pepper

Crumble and dissolve the chicken bouillon cubes in water and heat in a saucepan. In a skillet, heat the oil and sauté the onion and garlic for 3-4 minutes. Add the celery, finely chopped tomatoes, salt and pepper. Cook on low heat, stirring frequently for 10-15 minutes. Add the rice and continue heating for 20 minutes or until the rice is cooked. Remove from heat, add the fresh parsley and serve.

Note: Excellent source of Vitamin C. Good source of Vitamin A, B6, B1, Folate, Niacin and Iron.
Serving Size: 6
Prep Time: 0:40

Calories 158	Carbohydrate 30g	Cholesterol 0mg
Protein 4g	Fat 2g	Dietary Fiber 2g
	% Calories from fat 15%	

Root Vegetable Soup

- 2 carrots, peeled and diced
- 1 turnip, peeled and diced
- 1 rutabaga, peeled and diced
- 1 parsnip, peeled and diced
- 1 chopped onion
- 2 cloves crushed garlic
- 1 tablespoon parsley
- 1 tablespoon olive oil
- 3 cups water
- ¼ teaspoon sea salt
- ¼ teaspoon black pepper

Heat a large non-stick skillet and sauté the onion and garlic in olive oil. Add the turnip, rutabaga and parsnip and continue to sauté for 5 minutes. Add the carrot and sauté for 3 minutes. Add the water and bring to a boil. Cover and simmer for 30 minutes or until cooked. Adjust the seasonings and serve hot, garnished with fresh parsley.

Notes: Excellent source of Vitamin C, A and Folate. Good source of Vitamin B6 and B1. Half a cup of nonfat sour cream may be added to the cooked soup to increase the calcium content of the soup.
Serving Size: 4
Prep Time: 0:40

Calories 82	Carbohydrate 17g	Cholesterol 0mg
Protein 2g	Fat 1g	Dietary Fiber 5g
	% Calories from fat 14%	

Tomato Soup

- 12 medium tomatoes
- 1 large chopped onion
- 3 tablespoons tomato paste
- 3 cups chicken broth
- 1 teaspoon sugar
- ½ teaspoon pepper
- ½ teaspoon Tabasco sauce
- ½ teaspoon salt
- 1 teaspoon fresh basil

Combine the finely chopped and peeled tomatoes, onion, chicken broth and tomato paste in a large saucepan. Bring to a boil, reduce the heat, cover and simmer for 15-20 minutes. Cool and blend until smooth. Return to the pan, add the seasonings and heat through. Serve garnished with finely chopped fresh tomato.

Note: Excellent source of Vitamin C, A, Folate and Niacin. Good source of Vitamin B6, B1, B2 and Iron.
Serving Size: 6
Prep Time: 0:30

Calories 105	Carbohydrate 16g	Cholesterol 1mg
Protein 8g	Fat 2g	Dietary Fiber 3g
	% Calories from Fat 17%	

BEANS, PASTA AND RICE

Adzuki Beans and Rice

- 1 cup adzuki beans
- 1 medium onion
- 2 cloves garlic
- 1 teaspoon salt
- ¼ teaspoon chili powder
- 1 tablespoon olive oil
- 1 cup rice
- ½ cup vegetable broth

Wash beans and cover with water. Bring to a boil, remove from heat and let soak for one hour. Drain and add sufficient cold water to cover the beans. Add chopped onion, crushed garlic cloves and salt. Canned beans may be used. Bring to the boil and simmer for 1½ hours until tender. Add extra water if necessary. Place bean mixture in a blender and purée until smooth. Cook rice using broth as the liquid. Add chili powder to cooked rice and set aside. Heat olive oil in a heavy skillet and add puréed bean mixture. Simmer for 5 minutes, stirring frequently. Stir in rice and heat for a further 5 minutes. Serve with a fresh salad.

Notes: Excellent source of Vitamin B1, Folate, Niacin, Iron and Zinc. Good source of Vitamin A and B6.
Serves: 4
Prep Time: 2:00 hours (0:20)

Calories 390	Carbohydrate 73g	Cholesterol 0mg
Protein 14g	Fat 4g	Dietary Fiber 8g
	% Calories from fat 10%	

Baked Beans

3 cups pinto beans, canned	½ teaspoon mustard powder
1 large onion	1 teaspoon chili powder
1 can (15 ounces) tomato sauce	1 teaspoon honey

Preheat oven to 350°F. Chop onions and add to beans, tomatoes, onions, honey and seasonings. Bake in an oiled, uncovered casserole dish for an hour. This may be kept warm in a covered pot. Serve with hot bread and a mixed salad.

Optional: Add one cup chopped apple (with peel on).

Note: Excellent source of Folate. Good source of Vitamin C, A, B6, B1, B2, Iron and Zinc.

Serves: 4
Prep Time: 1:00 hour

Calories 174	Carbohydrate 34g	Cholesterol 0mg
Protein 10	Fat 2g	Dietary Fiber 8g
	% Calories from fat 4%	

Bean, Noodle and Nut Casserole

12 ounces noodles	4 medium onions
1 pound blackeyed peas	4 ounces cashews
½ tablespoon olive oil	4 ounces peanuts

Wash blackeyed peas. Boil 4 cups of water and drop the blackeyed peas in. Boil for 2 minutes. Set aside to soak for one hour. Cook noodles according to package instructions. Melt butter and sauté onions until clear and soft. Toss nuts with onions in the frying pan until browned lightly. Drain blackeyed peas and cover with 4 cups of cold water. Bring back to a boil and simmer for 30 minutes or until tender. Combine drained noodles, blackeyed peas, onions and nuts in a casserole dish. Cover and heat for 20 minutes in a 350° oven. Serve with tomato sauce and a fresh salad.

Notes: Excellent source of Vitamin B6, B12, B1, B2, Folate, Niacin, Iron and Zinc. Good source of Calcium. This is a satisfying vegetarian entree.

Serves: 10
Prep Time: 2:30 (20)
Reduce the prep time by 2 hours using canned beans.

Calories 429	Carbohydrate 59g	Cholesterol 0mg
Protein 21g	Fat 14g	Dietary Fiber 8g
	% Calories from Fat 28%	

Blackeyed Peas

- 2 quarts water
- 1 pound blackeyed peas
- 1 medium onion
- 1 teaspoon salt
- 1 red pepper pod, crushed
- 1 pound ground turkey
- 2 cloves garlic, crushed
- 1 teaspoon garlic powder
- 1 pinch baking soda

Bring water to boil. Add washed blackeyed peas, onion, garlic, salt, garlic powder and crushed red pepper pod. Cook on low heat until the peas are tender (about one hour). Mash the peas with a large wooden spoon then add ground turkey, ginger and baking soda. Adjust water to give a mushy consistency.

Note: Excellent source of Vitamin B6, B1, Folate, Niacin, Iron and Zinc. Good source of Vitamin C, B2 and Calcium.

Serves: 6
Prep Time: 1:30 (15)
Reduce the prep time by 1 hour by using canned peas

Calories 376	Carbohydrate 48g	Cholesterol 60mg
Protein 31g	Fat 7g	Dietary Fiber 8g
	% Calories from fat 17%	

Brown Rice Pilaf

- ¾ cup brown rice
- 2 cups vegetable broth
- 1 package frozen peas
- 1 chopped red bell pepper
- 1 medium chopped onion
- 3 cloves garlic, crushed
- 1 tablespoon olive oil

Heat the oil in a non-stick skillet. Sauté onions and garlic for 3-5 minutes. Add the brown rice and vegetable broth. Bring to a boil and boil for 5 minutes. Turn down the heat, cover the pan and simmer for 40 minutes. Check the level of liquid occasionally and add extra if necessary. Boil the peas and chopped peppers for 3 minutes and add the rice mixture. Mix thoroughly. Goes well with chicken or a bean dish.

Notes: Excellent source of Vitamin C, A, B6, B1, Folate and Iron. Good source of Vitamin B2, Niacin and Zinc. Optional extra for added protein: Add 1 cup diced chicken.

Serving Size: 6
Prep Time: 1:15

Calories 188	Carbohydrate 33g	Cholesterol 1mg
Protein 5g	Fat 4g	Dietary Fiber 2g
	% Calories from fat 20%	

Flageolets (Small French Green Beans)

- 2 cups flageolets, soaked
- 4 cups water
- 1 tablespoon olive oil
- 1 medium onion, chopped
- 2 cloves garlic, crushed
- ½ teaspoon salt
- ½ teaspoon black pepper
- 1 tablespoon parsley, chopped

Soak flageolets (beans) overnight. Drain and rinse. Heat the water in a pot. Heat the olive oil in a large skillet. Sauté the onion and garlic until lightly browned and soft (about 5 minutes). Stir in the drained flageolets and heat for 3 minutes over a low flame. Add the hot water and cover the pan. Simmer for one hour. Add extra water if necessary. Adjust seasoning and serve sprinkled with fresh, chopped parsley.

Note: Excellent source of Vitamin B1, Folate, Iron and Zinc. Good source of Vitamin B6 and Calcium.

Serves: 6
Prep Time: 1:30
Reduce prep time to 10 minutes by using canned beans.

Calories 228	Carbohydrate 42g	Cholesterol 0mg
Protein 13g	Fat 3g	Dietary Fiber 12g
	% Calories from fat 10%	

Lemon Rice

- 1½ cups long-grain rice
- 1½ cups water
- 2 tablespoons fresh lemon juice
- 1 tablespoon olive oil
- 1 tablespoon fresh parsley
- 1 medium onion, chopped fine
- ¼ teaspoon fresh dill

Heat a non-stick skillet and spray with olive oil. Sauté the onion for 2-3 minutes until transparent. Add the rice and dill. Cover with the water. Simmer covered for 20-30 minutes until cooked. Add the fresh lemon juice and season to taste. Serve garnished with parsley.

Serving Size: 4
Prep Time: 0:30

Calories 224	Carbohydrate 48g	Cholesterol 0mg
Protein 1g	Fat 3g	Dietary Fiber <1g
	% Calories from fat 14%	

Lentil and Pecan Casserole

- 2 cups lentils
- 1 tablespoon olive oil
- ¼ teaspoon thyme
- ½ cup pecans
- 1 teaspoon soy sauce
- 1 tablespoon cheddar cheese, shredded

Soak beans overnight in cold water. Drain and bring to the boil. Simmer until tender. Preheat the oven to 350°F. Crush the beans. Add chopped pecans and seasonings. Place in an oiled skillet. Heat for 15 minutes. Add grated cheese and continue heating until melted (3-5 minutes). Serve with a green salad.

Note: Excellent source of Vitamin B6, B1, Folate, Iron and Zinc. Good source of Vitamin C, B2 and Niacin.

Serves: 4

Prep Time: 2:00

Reduce prep time to 10 minutes by using canned lentils.

Calories 435	Carbohydrate 58g	Cholesterol 0mg
Protein 29g	Fat 12g	Dietary Fiber 30g
	% Calories from fat 24%	

Lentil Patties

- 1 cup lentils, canned
- 1 tablespoon olive oil
- 1 clove garlic
- ½ teaspoon salt
- 1 tablespoon liquid egg substitute or 1 egg
- ¼ teaspoon ground cumin
- ½ teaspoon curry powder
- 1 pinch celery salt
- ¾ cup bread crumbs

Preheat oven to 350°F. Stir lentils and seasonings together in a bowl. Add half of the bread crumbs. Lightly beat the egg with a fork and add to the mixture to bind (this step is optional). Using wet hands mold the lentil mixture into 8 evenly shaped patties. Place the remaining bread crumbs into a large plastic bag. Add the patties and roll them in the crumbs inside the bag until evenly covered. Remove the patties and set aside. Heat the olive oil in a skillet and lightly fry the patties to brown them. Place the skillet in the oven and bake for 20 minutes. Serve with a tomato or yogurt based sauce.

Note: Excellent source of Vitamin B6, B1, Folate and Iron. Good source of Vitamin B2, Niacin and Zinc.

Serves: 4

Prep Time: 0:30

Calories 303	Carbohydrate 44g	Cholesterol 53mg
Protein 18g	Fat 3g	Dietary Fiber 16g
	% Calories from fat 9%	

Mexican Bean Pie

- 4 corn tortillas
- ½ cup scallions, sliced thin
- 2 cloves garlic, crushed
- 2 green bell peppers, diced
- 1 tablespoon olive oil
- 2 cups pinto beans, cooked, mashed
- 2 tomatoes, chopped
- 2 teaspoons chili powder
- 1 teaspoon coriander ground
- ½ cup egg substitute, liquid
- ¼ cup cheddar cheese, shredded

Heat tortillas for 5-8 minutes over a flame or in a hot oven. Place in a blender or pestle and mortar and crumble finely. Take 4 pie pans (5" in diameter) and spray or coat with olive oil. Coat with the tortilla crumbs, setting aside extra for topping. Heat the rest of the olive oil in a heavy skillet and sauté the scallions, peppers and garlic for about 3-4 minutes, until tender. Add the beans, tomatoes, chili powder and coriander and continue to sauté for a further 5 minutes. Remove from the heat and stir in the egg substitute. Divide among the prepared pans and sprinkle the tops with the rest of the crumbs. Bake at 375°F for 20 minutes. Top with cheese and melt for a further few minutes in the hot oven. Serve with a salad.

Notes: Excellent source of Vitamin C, A, B6, B1, Folate and Iron. Good source of Vitamin B2, Calcium and Zinc.

Serves: 4
Prep Time: 0:45

Calories 281	Carbohydrate 41g	Cholesterol 2mg
Protein 15g	Fat 6g	Dietary Fiber 11g
	% Calories from fat 21%	

Navy Bean Stew

- ½ pound navy beans
- 2 tablespoons olive oil
- 1 large onion
- 1 clove garlic
- ½ cup tomato sauce
- 1 medium carrot
- 1 stalk celery
- ¼ teaspoon black pepper
- ¼ cup parsley sprigs
- 1 teaspoon dried basil
- 4 cups water

Soak rinsed and sorted navy beans in water overnight or use the short method by covering with 2 ½ cups of cold water, bringing to a boil for 2 minutes and then letting stand for one hour. Drain. Canned beans may be used. Heat olive oil in large soup pot and sauté chopped onions and crushed garlic clove until lightly browned and moist. Add tomato sauce, thinly sliced carrot, chopped celery, black pepper and simmer for 10 more minutes. Add navy beans and 4 cups of boiling water. Lower the heat and simmer in the covered pot until the beans are tender (about 45 minutes). Serve with hot bread or pasta salad for a nourishing main dish.

Note: Excellent source of Vitamin C, A, B6, B2, B1, Folate and Iron. Good source of Vitamin B2, Niacin, Calcium and Zinc.

Serves: 4
Prep Time: 0:15 (30)

Calories 279	Carbohydrate 41g	Cholesterol 0mg
Protein 14g	Fat 8g	Dietary Fiber 16g
	% Calories from fat 24%	

Noodles with Tuna

- 1 6 ounce can tuna in water
- 1 tablespoon fresh lemon juice
- ¾ pound linguini
- 4 quarts water
- ¼ teaspoon salt
- ¼ teaspoon black pepper
- 1 tablespoon virgin olive oil

Cook the pasta for 8-9 minutes until tender. Drain well and lay in a warm serving dish. While the pasta is cooking, prepare the tuna sauce. Drain the tuna and mix with the lemon juice and olive oil. Season to taste and set on top of the linguini. Sprinkle a little grated Parmesan or Romano cheese on the top.

Note: Excellent source of Vitamin B12, B1 and Niacin. Good source of Vitamin B2 and Iron.

Serving Size: 6
Prep Time: 0:45

Calories 322	Carbohydrate 43g	Cholesterol 8mg
Protein 14g	Fat 10g	Dietary Fiber 1g
	% Calories from fat 28%	

Pasta and Eggplant

- 2 tablespoons olive oil
- ½ lb fresh pasta
- 1 eggplant, peeled and chopped
- 4 cloves crushed garlic
- 28 ounces canned tomatoes
- ¼ teaspoon hot chili peppers
- ½ teaspoon salt
- ½ teaspoon black pepper
- 2 tablespoons fresh parsley
- 1 tablespoon grated Parmesan

Cook the pasta by boiling in salted water until tender. Meanwhile, heat one tablespoon of the oil in a large non-stick skillet and sauté the onion and garlic for 3-5 minutes. Add half of the eggplant and cook for 8-10 minutes until tender. Remove and keep warm. Heat the rest of the olive oil and cook the remainder of the eggplant. Add the tomatoes, chili peppers and seasoning. Return the eggplant to the pan and warm the whole mixture. Drain the pasta and serve with the sauce on top. Garnish with fresh parsley. Serve the Parmesan cheese separately.

Note: Excellent source of Vitamin C, A, B6, B1, B2, Folate, Niacin and Iron. Good source of Calcium and Zinc.

Serving Size: 4
Prep Time: 0:30

Calories 434	Carbohydrate 79g	Cholesterol 84mg
Protein 17g	Fat 7g	Dietary Fiber 5g
	% Calories from fat 14%	

Pasta Primavera

- 1 pound pea pods or mange tout
- 1 pound asparagus
- 1 cup green beans, sliced
- ½ cup carrots sliced thin
- 1 tablespoon olive oil
- ½ cup diced red bell pepper
- ½ cup diced yellow pepper
- 2 tablespoons chopped chives
- 4 tablespoons chopped parsley
- ¾ pound angel hair pasta

Bring a large pot of salted water to the boil. Blanch the pea pods, asparagus, green beans and carrots separately by dipping for 30 seconds and placing in ice cold water immediately afterwards for 30 seconds. Drain and pat dry. Save the cooking water. Heat the olive oil in a large skillet and sauté the bell peppers. Add the blanched vegetables and continue to heat for another 1-2 minutes. Re-boil the water and cook the pasta for 3-4 minutes, drain and transfer to a warm serving bowl. Add the hot vegetables and chives, toss and season to taste. Serve the pasta on individual pasta dishes and use fresh grated Parmesan cheese for topping.

Note: Excellent source of Vitamin C, A, B6, B1, B2, Folate, Niacin and Iron. Good source of Zinc.
Serving Size: 6
Prep Time: 0:40

Calories 296	Carbohydrate 55g	Cholesterol 0mg
Protein 12g	Fat 3g	Dietary Fiber 6g
	% Calories from fat 9%	

Quinoa-Nut Vegetable Pilaf

1 cup quinoa, rinsed and drained
1 tablespoon olive oil
1 medium chopped onion
1 clove crushed garlic
1 medium diced carrot
2 tablespoons almonds, toasted and chopped
2 tablespoons chopped parsley
1/2 teaspoon salt

Rinse the quinoa under cold running water for 4-5 minutes to remove the grit and bitter flavorings. Heat the olive oil in a large, non-stick pan and sauté the onion and garlic for 3-5 minutes until transparent. Add the carrot and continue to cook in the covered pan for 2-3 minutes more. Add the quinoa, water and salt and boil for 2 minutes. Reduce the heat, cover the pot and simmer for 20 minutes until tender. Add the chopped, toasted almonds and mix well. Add additional water if necessary so that the pilaf is moist. Serve hot.

Note: Excellent source of Vitamin A and Iron. Good source of Vitamin B6, B1, B2, Folate and Zinc.
Serving Size: 4
Prep Time: 1:00 hour

Calories 218	Carbohydrate 34g	Cholesterol 0mg
Protein 7g	Fat 6g	Dietary Fiber 4g
	% Calories from fat 25%	

Risotto

1 cup rice
1¾ cups vegetable broth
½ medium chopped onion
½ tablespoon extra virgin olive oil
1 teaspoon white wine

Heat the oil in a non-stick pan and sauté the onion and garlic for 3-4 minutes until transparent. Add the rice and vegetable broth and bring to a boil. Boil for a minute, then reduce the heat, cover the pan and simmer for 25 minutes or until tender. Add extra water if necessary. Serve hot.

Note: Excellent source of Vitamin A and B12. Good source of Niacin, Iron and Zinc.
Optional Extras: 1/2 teaspoon of powdered saffron or 1/2 cup of porcine mushrooms (sliced and sautéed with the onions and garlic).

Serving Size: 4
Prep Time: 0:40

Calories 260	Carbohydrate 49g	Cholesterol 1mg
Protein 6g	Fat 4g	Dietary Fiber 2g
	% Calories from fat 13%	

Spaghetti with Artichoke Hearts

- ¼ ounce can artichoke hearts
- 2 cloves crushed garlic
- 1 small chopped onion
- 2 tablespoons olive oil
- 3 tablespoons fresh chopped parsley
- ½ teaspoon basil
- ½ teaspoon salt
- ½ teaspoon black pepper
- ¼ cup grated Parmesan cheese
- 2 egg whites
- ¼ pound spaghetti

Rinse and quarter the canned artichoke hearts. Heat the olive oil in a skillet and sauté the onion and garlic for 3-4 minutes. Add ½ cup water, parsley, basil, salt and pepper. Simmer for 15 minutes. Boil a large pot of salted water and cook the spaghetti for 8-10 minutes or until cooked. Combine the egg whites and Parmesan cheese. Toss the pasta in the mixture. Add the artichoke mixture and reheat. Add extra water if it is too dry. Serve with extra Parmesan cheese as a topping.

Note: Excellent source of Vitamin C, B12, B2, Folate, Niacin and Iron. Good source of Vitamin B6, Calcium and Zinc.

Serving Size: 4
Prep Time: 0:30

Calories 355	Carbohydrate 56g	Cholesterol 4mg
Protein 14g	Fat 9g	Dietary Fiber 7g
	% Calories from fat 23%	

Southern Style Beans and Rice

- 1 cup canned red kidney beans
- 1 medium onion, chopped
- 1 small green bell pepper
- 1 pinch salt
- ¼ teaspoon black pepper
- ½ teaspoon Cajun seasoning
- 1 cup rice
- 1 Tablespoon olive oil

Drain and rinse the beans. Meanwhile cook the rice by covering with ½ inch of water and simmer in a covered pan until the water has been absorbed and the rice is cooked. Sauté the onion, garlic and chopped pepper for 6-8 minutes until browned and cooked. Add the beans and sufficient water to make a thick gravy. Season with the Cajun seasoning, salt and freshly ground black pepper. Serve with the rice.

Note: Excellent source of Vitamin C, B1 and Folate. Good source of Vitamin B6, Niacin, Iron and Zinc.

Serves: 6
Prep Time: 0:20

Calories 224	Carbohydrate 46g	Cholesterol 0mg
Protein 10g	Fat 1g	Dietary Fiber 6g
	% Calories from fat 2%	

Stir-fry Vegetables and Rice

- 1 medium chopped onion
- 1 peeled and chopped carrot
- 1 cup Mung bean sprouts
- 1 cup bok choy, sliced thick
- ¼ cup slivered almonds
- 2 tablespoons soy sauce
- ½ teaspoon black pepper
- ½ red bell pepper
- 2 sliced water chestnuts
- 1 teaspoon sesame oil
- 2 cups cooked brown rice

Heat the sesame oil in a large wok or deep skillet. Add the chopped onion and carrot and stir-fry for 2 minutes. Add the other vegetables and continue to stir-fry for 3-4 minutes more. Add the almonds, soy sauce and pepper. Serve with the cooked rice.

Note: Excellent source of Vitamin C, A, B6 and Folate. Good source of Vitamin B1, Niacin and Zinc.

Serving Size: 4
Prep Time: 0:10

Calories 210	Carbohydrate 33g	Cholesterol 0mg
Protein 6g	Fat 7g	Dietary Fiber 3g
	% Calories from fat 28%	

Tasty Rice and Tofu

- 1½ pounds tofu, low-fat
- ½ tablespoon olive oil
- 2 cloves crushed garlic
- 2 medium chopped onions
- 1 cup sliced mushrooms
- ½ cup Tamari soy sauce
- a dash Tabasco sauce
- 1 teaspoon fresh basil
- ½ teaspoon thyme
- ¼ teaspoon marjoram
- ¼ teaspoon savory
- 2 cups vegetable broth
- 2 cups cooked rice

Heat the olive oil in a nonstick skillet. Add the garlic and onions and sauté for 3-5 minutes until transparent. Add the mushrooms and cook 2 more minutes, shaking the skillet constantly. Remove the vegetables and set aside on a warm dish. Cut the tofu into 1 ½ inch size cubes. In a mixing bowl combine the Tamari, basil, thyme, savory, marjoram and Tabasco. Dip the tofu cubes in the mixture and brown the cubes in the skillet. Add the vegetable broth to the skillet and return the vegetable mixture. Simmer for 10 minutes and serve hot with rice as a main dish.

Note: Excellent source of Vitamin A and Iron. Good source of Vitamin B6, B1, B2, Folate, Niacin, Calcium and Zinc

Serving Size: 6
Prep Time: 0:20

FISH

Baked Red Snapper

- 4 pounds red snapper
- ½ tablespoon olive oil
- ½ tablespoon butter
- 1 medium chopped onion
- 3 sticks chopped celery
- 1 medium green bell pepper
- 4 cloves crushed garlic
- 1 teaspoon sugar
- 1 tablespoon Worcestershire sauce
- ¼ cup white wine
- 8 fluid ounces tomato sauce
- ½ teaspoon Creole seasoning
- 1 pinch salt
- 1 pinch black pepper, fresh ground

Season the fish and place in an ovenproof dish. Melt the olive oil and butter and sauté the onions, celery, green bell pepper and garlic for 5-8 minutes. Add the tomato sauce, Worcestershire sauce and season to taste. Cook slowly for one hour. Heat the oven to 300°F. Pour the wine over the fish and then the sauce. Place in the oven with a small piece of aluminum foil loosely on top. Cook for one hour, basting occasionally. Serve with rice or mashed potatoes as a main dish.

Note: Excellent source of Vitamin C and B12. Good source of Vitamin B6.

Serving Size: 8
Prep Time: 0:20
Baking Time: 2:00

Calories 85	Carbohydrate 6g	Cholesterol 18mg
Protein 10g	Fat 2g	Dietary Fiber 1g
	% Calories from fat 24%	

Baked Salmon

- 1 salmon (medium or 4-6 pounds)
- 1 medium sliced carrot
- 1 medium sliced onion
- 4 whole black peppercorns
- 1 sprig parsley
- 1 bay leaf

Place the salmon on a large piece of aluminum foil in an ovenproof dish. Slice the carrot and onion and arrange on top of the fish with the peppercorns, parsley and bay leaf. Dab with butter and wrap the foil around the fish. Add the water to the base of the dish and place in a cool oven (250°F) and cook for 2 to 3 hours until cooked through but not dry. Serve hot with Hollandaise Sauce, garnished with lemon wedges. Serve cold, garnished with thinly sliced cucumber, lemon slices and parsley. Cold salmon goes well with mayonnaise or a yogurt dressing.

Note: Excellent source of Vitamin C, A, B6, B12, Calcium and Iron. Good source of Niacin.

Serving Size: 8
Prep Time: 3:00 hours

Calories 355	Carbohydrate 2 g	Cholesterol 12 mg
Protein 45 g	Fat 14 g	Dietary Fiber <1g
	% Calories from fat 35%	

Barbecued Fish with Tarragon Sauce

2 medium red snapper
1 tablespoon fennel
1 tablespoon sage
2 bay leaves
1 tablespoon rosemary
½ tablespoon olive oil
1 tablespoon butter
4 tablespoons white wine
1 pinch salt
1 pinch black pepper

Tarragon Sauce

4 tablespoons tarragon
¼ cup butter substitute
1 cup lemon juice

Mix the finely chopped herbs except the tarragon together with the butter and place inside each fish. Brush the fish with oil and place in a wire fish barbecue griller. Grill over hot coals. Combine the ingredients for the tarragon sauce and warm in a small pan. Serve hot as a main dish.

Note: Excellent source of Vitamin C and B12. Good source of Vitamin A, B6, Calcium and Iron.
Serving Size: 4
Prep Time: 0:20

Calories 148	Carbohydrate 9.g	Cholesterol 28mg
Protein 10g	Fat 6g	Dietary Fiber <1g
	% Calories from fat 40%	

Broiled Orange Roughy

2 orange roughy fillets
6 medium tomatoes
1 medium red onion
2 cucumbers, peeled
1 teaspoon salt
2 tablespoons tarragon
1 teaspoon sugar
¼ cup red wine vinegar
½ tablespoon olive oil
½ teaspoon ground pepper
2 medium carrots, diced
¼ cup frozen green peas

Remove the core and seeds from the tomatoes and chop coarsely. Combine with the onion, cucumber, finely chopped tarragon, salt, sugar and chill. Season the orange roughy fillets with salt and fresh ground black pepper and brush (or spray) with olive oil. Broil for 2-3 minutes until cooked. At the same time place the diced carrots in a small saucepan and cover with cold water. Bring to the boil and simmer for 2 minutes. Add the frozen peas and continue to cook for another 2-3 minutes. Drain and set aside. Place the fish on a warm serving dish. Combine the peas and carrots with ½ cup of the chilled relish and arrange the vegetable mixture around the fish. Serve the rest of the relish as a side dish. Serve the fish hot with garlic mashed potatoes.

Note: Excellent source of Vitamin A, C, B6, B1, B2, Folate and Iron.
Serving Size: 2
Prep Time: 0:20

Calories 205	Carbohydrate 39g	Cholesterol 10mg
Protein 7g	Fat 5g	Dietary Fiber 9g
	% Calories from Fat 20%	

Creamy Dijon Sole

- 1 pound Dover sole fillets
- 1 small onion, chopped fine
- 4 tablespoons nonfat yogurt
- 2 tablespoons Dijon mustard
- 2 tablespoons olive oil
- 1 teaspoon fresh chopped tarragon

Preheat the oven to 425°F. Spray a shallow non-stick ovenproof dish with olive oil spray and arrange the onion slices in the pan. Place the fish over the onion slices. Combine the yogurt, mustard, olive oil and tarragon and season to taste with salt and pepper. Spread over the fish. Bake uncovered for 7-9 minutes. Serve hot with brown rice or small potatoes.

Notes: Good source of Niacin and Calcium. You can also use other white fish for this nutritious supper dish, low in calories and delicious. Fish is easy to digest and suitable for delicate stomachs.

Serving Size: 4
Prep Time: 0:15

Calories 158	Carbohydrate 3g	Cholesterol 0mg
Protein 19g	Fat 8g	Dietary Fiber 2g
	% Calories from fat 44%	

Ginger-Sesame Salmon

- 4 salmon steaks
- 1 teaspoon fresh lemon juice
- 1 cup water
- 2 teaspoons soy sauce
- 2 teaspoons rice vinegar
- 1 tablespoon fresh ginger root
- 2 green onions, cut in strips
- 1 clove garlic, crushed
- 1 tablespoon sesame oil

Place the water and fresh lemon juice in a deep non-stick sauté pan or skillet. Bring to a boil. Place the salmon steaks in the water and cover the pan. Reduce the heat and simmer very gently for 6-8 minutes until the fish is opaque in color. Arrange the salmon on a warm serving dish. Mix the soy sauce, rice vinegar and finely grated ginger together and spoon over the salmon. Cut the green onions into thin strips and scatter over the top of the fish. In a small pan combine the garlic and sesame oil. Warm the mixture until it browns and drizzle over the top of the fish. Serve hot.

Note: Excellent source of Vitamin C, B6, B12, B1, Folate and Niacin. Good source of Vitamin B2, Iron and Zinc.

Serving Size: 4
Prep Time: 0:20

Calories 254	Carbohydrate 6g	Cholesterol 88mg
Protein 36g	Fat 9g	Dietary Fiber 2g
	% Calories from fat 33%	

Grilled Tuna

- 4 medium tuna steaks
- ½ tablespoon olive oil
- a pinch of salt
- ¼ teaspoon black pepper

Brush the tuna steaks with olive oil and season with salt and pepper. Place a rack 4" from the broiler and heat for 10 minutes. Broil the steaks 4 minutes on each side. Serve on a bed of brown rice with warm cilantro sauce.

Note: Excellent source of Vitamin A, B6, B12, B1, B2 and Niacin.

Serving Size: 4
Prep Time: 0:20

Calories 260	Carbohydrate 1g	Cholesterol 65mg
Protein 40g	Fat 10g	Dietary Fiber 0g
	% Calories from fat 36%	

Halibut with Broccoli and Almonds

- ¾ pound halibut fillet
- 2 tablespoons corn starch
- ½ pound broccoli florets
- ½ cup julienned carrots
- ¼ cup low-sodium soy sauce
- 2 teaspoons sesame oil
- 1 clove garlic
- ½ teaspoon ginger
- 2 tablespoons almond slivers
- 2½ cups brown rice

Cut halibut into 1 inch by 2 inch strips and coat with corn starch. Combine broccoli, carrots, soy sauce, garlic and ginger in a mixing bowl and set aside. In a large non-stick skillet heat 2 teaspoons of sesame oil, add the fish and fry for 4 to 5 minutes until lightly browned. Remove the fish and set aside. Add the rest of the sesame oil and stir-fry the vegetable mixture for 3 to 4 minutes. Add the almonds and continue to cook for a further minute. Add the fish back to the mixture and warm through for one minute. Serve with the brown rice as a main dish.

Note: Excellent source of Vitamin C, A, B6, B12, B1, Folate, Niacin, Iron and Zinc. Good source of Vitamin B2 and Calcium.

Serving Size: 4
Prep Time: 0:20

Calories 590	Carbohydrate 101g	Cholesterol 27mg
Protein 30g	Fat 8g	Dietary Fiber 3g
	% Calories from fat 12%	

Monkfish, Mushrooms and Lentils

- 2 pounds monkfish
- 1 tablespoon flour
- 1 cup lentils
- 1 medium onion
- 2 tablespoons fresh parsley
- 2 cups porcini mushrooms
- 1½ cups water
- 2 teaspoons corn flour

1	bay leaf	½	cup white wine
1	leek	1	tablespoon olive oil
2	cloves garlic	1	tablespoon butter

Place the lentils and bay leaf in a pan with the water. Bring to a boil, cover and simmer for 20-30 minutes until the lentils are cooked. Set aside, still covered. Melt the oil and butter in a wide skillet. Add chopped onion, leek and garlic and sauté for 5 minutes. Add chopped parsley and continue to cook gently for a further 5 minutes. Add the porcini mushrooms and cook for 4-5 minutes more. Stir in the wine and cook for another minute. Add the filleted monkfish, dipped in seasoned flour. Simmer for 4 minutes on each side. Lift the fish out of the skillet and arrange on a large ovenproof dish. Cover and leave in a warm oven for 10 minutes. Mix 2 teaspoons of corn flour in 2 tablespoons of water and add to the skillet. Stir over a medium heat until the mixture thickens into a coating sauce. Serve the fish on a bed of lentils, covered with the porcini mushroom sauce.

Note: Excellent source of Vitamin B6, B1, B2, Folate, Niacin, Iron and Zinc. Good source of Vitamin C.

Serving Size: 4
Prep Time: 1:00

Calories 312	Carbohydrate 39g	Cholesterol 18mg
Protein 22g	Fat 8g	Dietary Fiber 7g
	% Calories from fat 22%	

Sea Bass with Apples

4	medium sea bass steaks	1	can tomatoes (15 ounces), chopped
2	medium red apples	½	cup vegetable broth
2	sticks celery, chopped	¼	teaspoon salt
2	medium onions, chopped	¼	teaspoon black pepper
4	teaspoons chopped parsley	1	pinch dill
1	medium green bell pepper, chopped		

Preheat the oven to 350°F. Place the celery, onions, tomatoes and broth into a pan and cook for 5 minutes. Core and dice the apple and add to the ingredients. Add the parsley and dill and season to taste. Continue cooking a further 2-3 minutes or until completely cooked. Place the mixture in the bottom of an ovenproof dish with the fish steaks on top. Cover with a loose piece of aluminum foil and bake in the oven at 350°F for 10-15 minutes until the fish is white and cooked. Garnish with parsley and lemon wedges. Serve hot with brown rice or mashed potato as a main dish.

Note: Excellent source of Vitamin C, A, B6, B1, Folate and Niacin. Good source of Calcium, Iron and Zinc.

Serving Size: 4
Prep Time: 0:30

Calories 233	Carbohydrate 24g	Cholesterol 53mg
Protein 27g	Fat 4g	Dietary Fiber 5g
	% Calories from fat 14%	

Sizzling Monkfish Broccoli and Peanuts

¾ pound monkfish (or other white fish)	1 clove garlic
2 tablespoons corn flour	1 teaspoon ground ginger
½ pound broccoli florets	1 teaspoon peanut oil
½ cup julienned carrots	1 tablespoon peanuts
¼ cup low-sodium soy sauce	2 ½ cups brown rice
½ teaspoon sesame oil	

Combine the fish, cut into 1 inch by 2 inch strips with the corn starch and cover evenly. In another bowl, combine the vegetables, sesame oil and seasoning. Heat 2 teaspoons of the peanut oil in a large skillet and add the fish, cooking until lightly browned (4-5 minutes). Remove the fish and set aside. Heat the remaining teaspoon of peanut oil and stir-fry vegetable mixture and peanuts. Cook for 4 minutes. Place the fish in the mixture and cook covered for another minute. Serve over steamed brown rice.

Note: Excellent source of Vitamin C, A, B6, B12, Folate and Niacin. Good source of Vitamin B1, B2, Iron and Zinc.

Serving Size: 4
Prep Time: 0:20

Calories 314	Carbohydrate 38g	Cholesterol 33mg
Protein 23g	Fat 7g	Dietary Fiber 3g
	% Calories from fat 22%	

Teriyaki Salmon

2 pounds salmon	1 teaspoon all-purpose flour
1 tablespoon brown sugar	½ cup white wine
¼ cup soy sauce	1 teaspoon mustard
1 tablespoon olive oil	6 slices pineapple

Combine soy sauce, brown sugar, olive oil, flour, wine and mustard in a small pan. Bring to a boil, and then simmer for 3 minutes. Set aside to cool. Wipe fish and pat dry. Preheat the oven to 320°F. Place the fish in the marinade and refrigerate for 15 minutes. Remove the fish from the refrigerator and place on a non-stick oiled pan. Place a slice of pineapple on each fillet. Heat the marinade and brush the fish with hot marinade. Place in the oven for 15 to 20 minutes until white and cooked. Remove and serve garnished with tomatoes for color. Serve with rice as a main dish.

Note: Excellent source of Vitamin C, B6, B12, B1, B2, Folate, Niacin and Iron.

Serving Size: 8
Prep Time: 0:45

Calories 198	Carbohydrate 7g	Cholesterol 62mg
Protein 24g	Fat 9g	Dietary Fiber 0.5g
	% Calories from fat 23%	

Trout with Almonds

- 4 trout
- ¼ cup almond slivers
- ¼ cup flour
- ½ tablespoon butter
- ½ tablespoon olive oil
- 1 lemon
- ¼ teaspoon salt
- ¼ teaspoon black pepper

Roll each prepared trout in the seasoned flour. Heat the oil and butter in a large non-stick skillet. Fry the trout 3-4 minutes on each side. Lift from the pan and set aside in a warm place. Add the almonds to the pan, adding extra oil and butter only if absolutely necessary. When browned, lift from the heat and set aside with the fish. Remove the skillet from the heat and add the lemon juice. Mix well and spoon the almonds and juices over the fish. Serve hot as a main dish.

Note: Excellent source of Vitamin C, B12, B1 and B2. Good source of Iron.

Serving Size: 4
Prep Time: 0:30

Calories 268	Carbohydrate 11g	Cholesterol 65mg
Protein 21g	Fat 12g	Dietary Fiber <1g
	% Calories from fat 47%	

White Fish with Ginger and Lemon

- 4 medium halibut steaks
- 2 tablespoons olive oil
- 2 garlic cloves
- 3 cups frozen green peas
- 2 sliced scallions
- 1 teaspoon peeled chopped ginger root
- 1 tablespoon grated lemon peel
- 1 cup lemon juice
- 2 cups cooked brown rice

Heat one tablespoon of the olive oil in a large nonstick skillet. Sauté the fish steaks until they turn white. Remove the fish and set aside in a warm place. Add the rest of the oil, peas, scallions, ginger and lemon peel. Cook, stirring frequently until the peas are cooked. Return the fish to the pan and heat thoroughly. Serve on a bed of brown rice. Garnish with lemon wedges and parsley. Serve as a main dish.

Note: Excellent source of Vitamin C, A, B6, B12, B1, Folate, Niacin and Iron. Good source of Vitamin B2, Calcium and Zinc.

Serving Size: 4
Prep Time: 0:20

Calories 460	Carbohydrate 45g	Cholesterol 54mg
Protein 44g	Fat 11g	Dietary Fiber 6g
	% Calories from fat 23%	

POULTRY

Chicken Curry

- 6 chicken breast halves, skinless
- 6 teaspoons curry powder

1½ cups chicken broth
5 teaspoons Worcestershire sauce
5 crushed bay leaves
½ teaspoon Tabasco sauce
3 teaspoons oregano
1 teaspoon paprika
2 cloves crushed garlic

Preheat the oven to 350°F. Combine all the ingredients except the chicken breasts in a pan and bring to the boil. Place the chicken in an ovenproof dish and cover with the mixture. Bake 50 minutes in covered dish. Note: Excellent source of Vitamin B6 and Niacin.

Serving Size: 6
Prep Time: 0:10
Baking Time: 0:50

Calories 139	Carbohydrate 4g	Cholesterol 52mg
Protein 24g	Fat 3g	Dietary Fiber 1g
	% Calories from fat 17%	

Chicken in Soy Sauce

4 skinless chicken legs
1 cup soy sauce
2 tablespoons honey
1 clove crushed garlic
4 green onions sliced diagonally

Combine the soy sauce, honey and garlic. Marinate the chicken legs for at least 2 hours or overnight. Bake in a covered dish for one hour at 350°F. Serve with rice or mashed potatoes. Sprinkle with onions.

Note: Excellent source of Vitamin B6, B2 and Niacin. Good source of Vitamin B1 and Folate

Serving Size: 4
Prep Time: 1:00
Marinate Time: 2:00+

Calories 234	Carbohydrate 14g	Cholesterol 113mg
Protein 32g	Fat 5g	Dietary Fiber <1g
	% Calories from fat 21%	

Chicken with Tarragon

2 pounds chicken, skinless
1½ tablespoon butter
½ tablespoon olive oil
4 sprigs fresh tarragon
½ teaspoon salt
½ teaspoon black pepper
1 clove crushed garlic

Preheat the oven to 325°F. Crush the garlic into the butter and oil and mix together. Smear this mixture over the breasts of the chicken. Place one sprig of tarragon inside each of the pieces and place them in a baking dish. Cover with a piece of aluminum foil leaving the sides open. Place in the oven for 20 minutes, turning twice. Remove the foil and brown for 5 more minutes or until cooked. Serve with a green salad.

Note: Excellent source of Vitamin B6 and Niacin. Good source of Vitamin B2 and Iron.

Serving Size: 4
Prep Time: 0:30

Calories 166	Carbohydrate 2g	Cholesterol 70mg
Protein 27g	Fat 5g	Dietary Fiber <1g
	% Calories from fat 28%	

Lemon Chicken and English Walnuts

- 4 chicken breast halves, skinless
- 2 tablespoons fresh lemon juice
- 2 tablespoons chopped walnuts
- 2 tablespoons soy sauce
- 1 tablespoon corn flour
- ¼ teaspoon white pepper

Preheat the oven to 325°F. Dissolve the corn flour in the soy sauce and lemon juice. Add the white pepper and chopped walnuts. Heat a non-stick skillet sprayed with olive oil and add the chicken breast halves. Brown for 2-3 minutes on each side. Remove and set aside on a warm serving dish. Add the sauce and allow the corn flour to thicken. Adjust the consistency if desired. Pour over the chicken and place in oven for 20 minutes. Serve hot.

Note: Excellent source of Vitamin B6 and Niacin. Good source of Vitamin B1 and Zinc.

Serving Size: 4
Prep Time: 0:10
Baking Time: 0:20

Calories 166	Carbohydrate 5g	Cholesterol 65mg
Protein 27g	Fat 4g	Dietary Fiber <1g
	% Calories from fat 21%	

Oven-baked Sesame Chicken

- 4 chicken breasts, skinless
- ½ cup flour
- ¼ cup sesame seeds
- ¼ teaspoon garlic powder
- ¼ teaspoon black pepper
- ½ teaspoon paprika
- ½ teaspoon salt
- ¼ cup 1% low-fat milk

Toast sesame seeds in a skillet until golden brown, stirring constantly. Preheat the oven to 400°F. Lightly oil a shallow baking pan. Combine flour, sesame seeds, garlic powder, black pepper, paprika and salt in a bag and shake well. Dip the chicken in milk and then coat in the bag. Place chicken in baking pan and bake for 45 minutes until golden brown.

Note: Excellent source of Vitamin B6, B1 and Niacin. Good source of Vitamin B2, Folate and Zinc.

Serving Size: 4
Prep Time: 0:10
Baking Time: 0:45

Calories 243	Carbohydrate 14g	Cholesterol 66mg
Protein 31g	Fat 7g	Dietary Fiber <1g
	% Calories from fat 25%	

VEGETABLES AND VEGETARIAN DISHES

Brussels Sprouts and Chestnuts

2 cups Brussels sprouts (small size are tastiest)
½ cup roasted chestnuts (fresh or canned)

Steam Brussels sprouts until just tender (8-10 minutes). Place on a serving dish and arrange warmed roasted chestnuts on top. Serve with roast turkey or chicken.

Note: Excellent source of Vitamin A, C and Folate. Good source of Vitamin B6.
Serving Size: 4
Prep Time: 0:15

Calories 62	Carbohydrate 13g	Cholesterol 0mg
Protein 2g	Fat <1g	Dietary Fiber 4g
	% Calories from fat 7%	

Eggplant Parmesan

3 medium eggplants, thinly sliced
1 chopped red bell pepper
1 tablespoon olive oil
1 clove crushed garlic
2 medium chopped onions
1 pound shredded carrots
1 pound mushrooms
½ small can black olives, sliced
1 can (15 ounces) tomatoes
6 ounces tomato paste
1½ teaspoons oregano
1 cup mozzarella cheese
1½ cups Ricotta cheese
1 tablespoon, Parmesan
1 cup chopped parsley
1½ cups bread crumbs
1 teaspoon black pepper

Preheat the oven to 350°F. Sprinkle salt on the eggplant slices and set aside for 20 minutes. Heat the oil in non-stick skillet and sauté the onions and garlic for 3 minutes or until transparent. Add the mushrooms and heat for 2 minutes. Add the shredded carrots and red pepper and cook for 2 minutes more while stirring. Add the tomatoes, tomato paste, olives and oregano. Season to taste and set aside. Drain and wipe dry the eggplant slices. Lay them in a large oiled ovenproof dish and add a layer of mozzarella and ricotta cheese, then a layer of the vegetable mixture. Repeat once more and finally sprinkle with Parmesan cheese. Place in the oven and bake for 45 minutes.

Note: Excellent source of Vitamin C, A, B6, B1, B2, Folate, Niacin, Calcium, Iron and Zinc.
Serving Size: 8

Prep Time: 1:15 hours

Calories 336	Carbohydrate 48g	Cholesterol 23mg
Protein 19g	Fat 10g	Dietary Fiber 10g
	% Calories from fat 25%	

Fennel Ratatouille

- 2 fennel bulbs
- 1 pound red ripe tomatoes
- 2 medium sliced onions
- 2 sliced zucchini
- 2 tablespoons fresh chopped parsley
- ½ teaspoon fresh thyme
- ¼ teaspoon salt
- ¼ teaspoon black pepper
- ½ tablespoon extra virgin olive oil

Heat the olive oil in a non-stick skillet and sauté the onions and garlic for 3-4 minutes until transparent. Add the fennel bulbs cut into slices, layered with zucchini and tomatoes. Sprinkle with herbs and season to taste. Cover the skillet and cook slowly for approximately an hour or until the fennel is tender. Serve hot or cold, garnished with chopped parsley.

Note: Excellent source of Vitamin C, A and Folate. Good source of Vitamin B6, B1, Niacin, Calcium and Iron.

Serving Size: 4
Prep Time: 1:10 hours

Calories 100	Carbohydrate 19g	Cholesterol 0mg
Protein 4g	Fat 2g	Dietary Fiber 3g
	% Calories from fat 19%	

French Peas

- 2 cups green peas
- ½ cup small white onions
- ½ teaspoon butter (optional)

Boil ½ cup of water and add green peas. Simmer for 5-8 minutes until cooked. Add onions and keep warm with pan covered. Add seasoning to taste. Add butter for optional shiny appearance.

Note: Excellent source of Vitamin C and Folate. Good source of Vitamin B1.

Serving Size: 4
Prep Time: 0:10

Calories 62	Carbohydrate 11g	Cholesterol 0mg
Protein 4g	Fat <1g	Dietary Fiber 4g
	% Calories from fat 4%	

Frittata with Spinach

- 2 eggs
- ¼ teaspoon red pepper flakes (optional)

2 egg whites	½ tablespoon extra virgin olive oil
½ teaspoon salt	½ cup grated Parmesan
1 clove garlic	1 pound spinach leaves, chopped fine
1 teaspoon paprika	

Preheat the oven to 350°F. Place the washed spinach in a large saucepan and cook covered for 3-4 minutes, shaking frequently. Drain well. Beat the eggs together (or use 1 ½ cups of liquid egg substitute) and add half of the eggs to the chopped spinach. Mix in 1/4 cup of the grated Parmesan. Prepare an 8 inch round oven-proof dish by lightly brushing with oil. Pour the egg and spinach mixture into the dish and sprinkle with the red pepper flakes. Pour the rest of the egg mixture over this and sprinkle with the rest of the Parmesan and paprika. Bake for 45 minutes and serve hot with a green salad as a main dish.

Note: Excellent source of Vitamin C, A, B2, Folate, Calcium and Iron. Good source of Zinc.

Serving Size: 4
Prep Time: 1:00 hour

Calories 134	Carbohydrate 5g	Cholesterol 114 mg
Protein 12 g	Fat 7 g	Dietary Fiber 3g
	% Calories from fat 49%	

Garlic Mashed Potatoes

4 peeled potatoes	1 teaspoon butter
½ cup skim milk	¼ teaspoon sea salt
3 cloves crushed garlic	¼ teaspoon black pepper

Heat the oven to 425°F. Wrap the garlic cloves in aluminum foil and bake for 20 minutes. Unwrap and cool. Slice the potatoes evenly and place in a saucepan. Cover with cold water and bring to a boil. Simmer for 5-8 minutes until soft. Drain and mash until smooth. Cut the base from the garlic cloves and squeeze pulp into mashed potatoes. Warm milk and add to potatoes with butter and seasonings. Serve hot or cold.

Note: Excellent source of Vitamin C. Good source of Vitamin B6 and Niacin.

Serving Size: 4
Prep Time: 0:30

Calories 111	Carbohydrate 23g	Cholesterol 3mg
Protein 4g	Fat 1g	Dietary Fiber 2g
	% Calories from fat 9%	

Glazed Carrots

5 medium carrots	½ tablespoon fresh lemon juice
½ tablespoon butter	1 tablespoon chopped parsley

Peel and julienne the carrots into ¼ inch long strips. Place them in a medium saucepan and cover with cold water. Bring to a boil and boil gently for 10-12 minutes or until tender. Drain and set aside in a warm place. In the same pan, melt butter and add lemon juice. Add carrots and toss for 1-2 minutes until well glazed.

Serve hot, garnished with fresh chopped parsley.

Note: Excellent source of Vitamin A. Good source of Vitamin C.
Serving Size: 4
Prep Time: 0:30

Calories 52	Carbohydrate 10g	Cholesterol 4mg
Protein 1g	Fat 1g	Dietary Fiber 3g
	% Calories from fat 17%	

Leeks a la Grécque

- 4 medium leeks
- 1 tablespoon olive oil
- 1 cup water
- 1 tablespoon tomato paste
- 1 teaspoon sugar
- ½ cup rice
- 12 small black olives
- 1 tablespoon parsley
- 1 teaspoon lemon juice
- 3 slices lemon

Wash and slice leeks into 1 ½ inch pieces. Steam for 5-6 minutes until cooked. Cool. Boil water, oil, tomato paste and sugar in a large pan and simmer for 5 minutes. Add rice, cover the pot and simmer for 8 minutes or until the liquid is completely absorbed by the rice. Turn off the heat and leave the pan covered for 10 minutes. Add lemon juice and arrange with leeks on a serving dish. Garnish with olives, parsley and lemon slices.

Note: Excellent source of Vitamin C, B6, B1, Folate and Iron. Good source of Niacin and Calcium.
Serving Size: 4
Prep Time: 0:30

Calories 229	Carbohydrate 48g	Cholesterol 0mg
Protein 5g	Fat 5g	Dietary Fiber 3g
	% Calories from fat 19%	

Potatoes au Gratin

- 2 pounds peeled potatoes
- 2 cups skim milk
- 4 tablespoons Swiss cheese
- 2 tablespoons Parmesan
- ¼ teaspoon salt
- ¼ teaspoon white pepper

Place the sliced potatoes in cold water and leave for 5 minutes. Drain and place in an ovenproof gratin dish. Add milk and season to taste with salt and pepper. Cover with foil and place in a medium hot oven (325°F) for 20 minutes. Add grated cheeses and return to the oven for 20-30 minutes or until the potatoes are cooked through. Serve hot.

Note: Excellent source of Vitamin C, B12 and Calcium. Good source of Vitamin B6 and B2.
Serving Size: 4
Prep Time: 0:30

Calories 111	Carbohydrate 17g	Cholesterol 7mg
Protein 8g	Fat 1g	Dietary Fiber <1g
	% Calories from fat 11%	

Sautéed Spinach

- 2 pounds fresh washed spinach
- 1 clove crushed garlic
- 1 tablespoon sesame oil
- ¼ teaspoon salt
- ¼ teaspoon black pepper

Place the washed spinach in a large saucepan and cook covered for 3-4 minutes, shaking frequently. Drain well. Heat the sesame oil in a large skillet and add the crushed garlic. Quickly stir-fry the spinach in the garlic and sesame oil and serve hot.

Note: Excellent source of Vitamin A and Folate. Good source of Vitamin C.

This dish is so low in calories that the % of fat calories seems high. The fat source is healthy oils which don't need to be restricted and can provide satiety.

Serving Size: 4
Prep Time: 0:10

Calories 38	Carbohydrate 1g	Cholesterol 0mg
Protein <1g	Fat 3g	Dietary Fiber 1g
	% Calories from fat 71%	

Spinach, Brown Rice and Tofu

- 1 cup brown rice
- 12 ounces tofu, firm
- 2 pounds spinach leaves
- 1 tablespoon soy sauce
- 1 tablespoon olive oil
- 1 tablespoon sesame seeds

Cook brown rice by covering in cold water with about 1/2 inch extra water on top. Bring to a boil and boil for a minute. Cover, turn the heat down and simmer for 30 - 40 minutes. Check the moisture level twice during cooking and adjust if necessary. Toast the sesame seeds for a few minutes in a medium oven (350° F). Wash and cook spinach in water by shaking a covered pot over a medium heat for 3-5 minutes. Arrange tofu in the middle of an ovenproof dish with spinach around the outside. Moisten with soy sauce and sprinkle the sesame seeds. Warm through in 325 degree oven and serve with rice.

Note: Excellent source of Vitamin C, A, B6, Folate and Iron. Good source of Vitamin B1, B2, Niacin, Calcium and Zinc.

Serving Size: 8
Prep Time: 0:45

Calories 164	Carbohydrate 22g	Cholesterol 0mg
Protein 10g	Fat 4g	Dietary Fiber 4g

% Calories from fat 23%

Sweet and Sour Vegetables

- 2 cups sliced carrots
- 2 cups chopped bok choy
- 2 cups chopped green bell pepper
- 3 cups chopped tomatoes
- 1 cup chopped onions
- 2 tablespoons tomato paste
- ¼ cup soy sauce
- ½ cup pineapple juice
- 1 can sliced water chestnuts
- 1 tablespoon corn starch

Steam the carrots till tender, add the bok choy and green peppers. Set aside. Dissolve the corn starch in the pineapple juice. Place the soy sauce, water and tomato paste in a small pan. Add the corn starch and pineapple mixture and bring to the boil. Stir well until it thickens. Sauté the onions in a covered, heavy bottom pan. Add the water chestnuts and the other vegetables and warm through. Add the sauce and serve in a dish with rice or pasta as a main dish.

Note: Excellent source of Vitamin C, A, B6 and Niacin. Good source of Vitamin B1 and Niacin.

Serving Size: 6
Prep Time: 0:45

Calories 76	Carbohydrate 17g	Cholesterol 0mg
Protein 3g	Fat <1g	Dietary Fiber 4g
	% Calories from fat 6%	

Sweet Potatoes with Almonds

- 2 pounds sweet potatoes or yams
- 1 tablespoon slivered almonds

Preheat the oven to 400° F. Toast the slivered almonds for 3-4 minutes until brown. Remove and set aside to cool. Bake the sweet potatoes for 20-30 minutes until soft. (They can also be baked in the microwave oven). When cool, split open and scoop out the center. Mash, adding a little water if necessary. Spread in a serving dish and cover with toasted slivered almonds.

Note: Excellent source of Vitamin C and A. Good source of Vitamin B6.

Serving Size: 4
Prep Time: 0:30

Calories 82	Carbohydrate 16g	Cholesterol 0mg
Protein 2g	Fat <1g	Dietary Fiber 2g
	% Calories from fat 15%	

Vegetable Curry

- 4 cups brown rice

Sauce

- 1½ cups cauliflower florets
- 2 tablespoons olive oil

2	medium carrots, sliced thin	1	tablespoon curry powder
1	cup broccoli florets	2	cloves garlic
1	medium red bell pepper, sliced	½	cup vegetable broth
¼	teaspoon red chili pepper or cayenne	2	tablespoons fresh lime juice
1	medium onion, sliced thin	1	cup frozen green peas
1	can (15 ounces) tomatoes	1	tablespoon toasted bread crumbs

Cook rice by covering with an extra half inch of water on top. Bring to a boil and boil for a minute uncovered. Cover the pot and simmer gently for 30 minutes. Check water level and adjust so that all water is absorbed and the rice is moist when cooked. Steam the cauliflower, sliced carrots and broccoli for 7-8 minutes, then add the red bell pepper, sliced onion and green peas and steam 3 minutes more. Add the tomatoes at the last minute and mix. Set aside in a casserole dish. Heat oil in a non-stick pan and add curry powder, garlic and red chili pepper. Sauté for 2-3 minutes. Add vegetable broth and boil for 3 minutes. Stir in fresh lime juice and pour over the vegetables. Sprinkle the top with toasted bread crumbs and serve hot.

Notes: Excellent source of Vitamin A, B6, B1, Folate, Niacin and Zinc. Good source of Vitamin B2 and Iron. Curry powder varies in intensity according to the brand. Start with a small amount and add extra to taste. The flavor will intensify as the dish stands.

Serving Size: 8
Prep Time: 0:30

Calories 434	Carbohydrate 86g	Cholesterol 0mg
Protein 11g	Fat 7g	Dietary Fiber 4g
	% Calories from fat 13%	

Vegetarian Stew

1	cup cooked brown rice	1	can (15 ounces) tomatoes
¾	cup bulgur	1	can (12 ounces) corn, drained
¾	cup cooked soybeans	1	teaspoon olive oil
½	pound sliced string beans	1	small can green chilies, drained
1	teaspoon chili powder	½	teaspoon black pepper
½	teaspoon hot sauce		

Soak the soybeans overnight and discard the water. Cook the brown rice by covering with ½ inch of cold water and bringing to a boil. Reduce heat, cover pot and simmer for 30 minutes or until tender. Cook the bulgur wheat in a similar manner in a separate pot. Drain the cans of chilies and corn. Heat the olive oil and add rice, bulgur, and soybeans. Quickly sauté until well mixed. Add string beans, corn, tomatoes and chilies. Season with chili powder and hot sauce. Add pepper. Simmer for 15 minutes. Serve hot.

Note: Excellent source of Vitamin C and Folate. Good source of Vitamin A, B6, B1, B2, Niacin and Iron.

Serving Size: 8
Prep Time: 0:45

Calories 210	Carbohydrate 41g	Cholesterol 0mg
Protein 8g	Fat 3g	Dietary Fiber 5g
	% Calories from fat 12%	

Vegetarian Tofu

1½ pounds low-fat tofu, firm
½ tablespoon olive oil
2 cloves crushed garlic
2 medium chopped onions
1 cup sliced mushrooms
¾ cup Tamari soy sauce
1 teaspoon fresh chopped basil
½ teaspoon thyme
¼ teaspoon marjoram
¼ teaspoon savory
a dash Tabasco sauce
2 cups vegetable broth
2 cups cooked brown rice

Heat the olive oil in a non-stick skillet. Add the garlic and onions and sauté for 3-5 minutes until transparent. Add the mushrooms and cook 2 more minutes, shaking the skillet constantly. Remove the vegetables and set aside on a warm dish. Cut the tofu into 1- 1 ½ inch size cubes. In a mixing bowl combine the Tamari, basil, thyme, savory, marjoram and Tabasco. Dip the tofu cubes in the mixture and brown the cubes in the skillet. Add the vegetable broth to the skillet and return the vegetable mixture. Simmer for 10 minutes and serve hot with rice as a main dish.

Note: Excellent source of Vitamin A and Iron. Good source of Vitamin B6, B1, B2, Folate, Niacin, Calcium and Zinc.

Serving Size: 6
Prep Time: 0:45

Calories 231	Carbohydrate 33g	Cholesterol 1mg
Protein 12g	Fat 6g	Dietary Fiber 3g
	% Calories from fat 23%	

DESSERTS AND COMFORT FOODS

Angel Food Cake

1½ cups flour, cake, sifted
1¾ cups sugar
14 egg whites
¼ teaspoon salt
2 teaspoons vanilla extract
1 teaspoon fresh lemon juice

Preheat the oven to 300°F. Beat the egg whites (which should be at room temperature) until fluffy but not dry. Fold the sugar with a metal spoon into the egg whites and then lightly fold in the sifted flour. Add the vanilla extract and lemon juice. Pour into an 8 inch diameter cake pan or a 10 inch tube pan. Smooth the top and place in the middle of the oven. Bake until a pale color and the top is spongy. A toothpick should come out clean. Cool in the pan and remove to place on a serving dish by releasing with a palette knife. Serve with fresh fruit and nonfat yogurt or ice cream.

Note: Good source of Vitamin B1 and B2.

Serves: 10
Prep Time: 0:20
Baking time: 0:30

Calories 219	Carbohydrate 48g	Cholesterol 0mg
Protein 6g	Fat <1g	Dietary Fiber <1g
	% Calories from fat <1%	

Apricot Almond Squares

- 1 cup dried apricot halves
- ½ cup dry roast almonds, ground
- 2 tablespoons butter
- ¼ cup of oatmeal
- ¼ cup sugar
- 1 teaspoon vanilla extract
- ½ teaspoon almond extract
- ½ teaspoon salt
- 1 cup flour
- ½ cup egg substitute, liquid
- 1 cup light brown sugar
- ½ teaspoon baking powder
- 1 tablespoon confectioner's sugar

Preheat the oven to 350ºF. Place apricots in a pan of cold water and bring to a boil. Cover and simmer for 6-8 minutes. Drain and pat dry. Slice thinly, cover and set aside. Blend the butter and oatmeal with 2 tablespoons water. Mix in half of the flour and the ground almonds with a metal spoon. Spread over the bottom of a 9 inch baking pan. Bake for 20 minutes. While the pastry is baking, sift the rest of the flour with the baking powder and salt. Lightly beat the egg substitute with the brown sugar and blend in the flour mixture. Add the vanilla and almond extracts and stir in the apricots. Spread over the pastry. Bake for 30 minutes until brown. Cool and sift confectioner's sugar over the squares before serving.

Note: This makes a wonderful base for fresh berries and can be prepared in advance

Serves: 36
Prep Time: 0:10
Baking time: 0:50

Calories 67	Carbohydrate 13g	Cholesterol 0mg
Protein 1g	Fat 1g	Dietary Fiber 1g
	% Calories from fat 15%	

Apricot and Strawberry Cake

- 2¾ cups flour
- 2½ teaspoons baking powder
- 1¾ cups sugar
- 1¼ cups skim milk
- ¾ cup apricots, puréed
- 2 eggs, beaten
- 1½ teaspoons vanilla
- 9 tablespoons strawberry jam
- 8 large strawberries, sliced thin
- 2 tablespoons apricot brandy glaze

Preheat the oven to 375ºF. Sift the flour, baking powder and sugar in a mixing bowl and stir to blend. Using a metal spoon combine the skim milk, apricot purée, eggs and vanilla with the dry ingredients. Pour the batter into two 8" cake pans sprayed with oil. Bake for 25 - 30 minutes or until a toothpick comes out dry from the center. Let the cake cool in the pan for 5 minutes before removing and cooling on a rack. Split each cake in half horizontally and fill with strawberry preserves. Brush the apricot brandy glaze (or apricot glaze) on the top and arrange strawberry slices in a petal-shaped pattern on the top. Glaze the strawberry slices also and serve with fresh whipped cream; low or nonfat yogurt or ice cream.

Note:: Excellent source of Vitamin C, B1 and B2. Good source of Vitamin A, Folate, Niacin, Calcium and Iron. Good source of Vitamin A, B6 and Zinc.

Serves: 8
Prep Time: 0:10
Baking time: 0:35

Calories 465	Carbohydrate 106g	Cholesterol 54mg
Protein 9g	Fat 2g	Dietary Fiber 4g
	% Calories from fat 4%	

Banana Bread

- 2 medium bananas
- 3 egg whites
- 2 tablespoons canola oil
- ½ teaspoon cinnamon
- ½ teaspoon nutmeg
- 1 tablespoon honey
- 1½ cups flour
- 2 teaspoons baking powder
- ½ teaspoon salt

Preheat the oven to 350°F. Lightly grease a 9 X 5 loaf pan. Beat the egg whites until fluffy, but not dry. Mash the bananas with the honey and canola oil and fold into the egg whites. In another bowl, sift the flour and salt. Add the baking powder, ground cinnamon and ground nutmeg. Combine with the banana mixture using light, firm strokes. Place the batter into the loaf pan and bake for 50 to 60 minutes or until a toothpick comes out clean. Cool for 10 minutes before turning out. Slice and serve warm or cold.

Note: Good source of Vitamin B1. Variations: Add 8 apricot halves, finely chopped OR 1/2 cups golden raisins OR 1/3 cup pecans or English walnuts, chopped.

Serves: 10
Prep Time: 0:10
Baking time: 1:00

Calories 121	Carbohydrate 22g	Cholesterol 0mg
Protein 2g	Fat 3g	Dietary Fiber 1g
	% Calories from fat 22%	

Ginger Cookies

- ½ cup apple sauce
- 1 cup butter
- 1¾ cups sugar
- ¾ cup brown sugar
- 1 medium egg
- 1¼ teaspoons baking soda
- 10½ teaspoons cinnamon
- 2 tablespoons ginger
- 1 tablespoon cloves
- 1 tablespoon nutmeg

½ cup molasses	½ teaspoon salt
2 ¾ cups white flour	½ cup powdered sugar

Preheat the oven to 350°F. Cream butter and sugar together until light and fluffy, taking about 8 to 10 minutes by hand or 4 to 5 minutes in a food processor. Lightly fold in the beaten egg and molasses. Sift flour, baking soda and salt and lightly fold into the mixture with firm strokes using a metal spoon. Season with the cinnamon, ginger, cloves, nutmeg and salt. Form ¾ inch round balls of dough, flatten a little and dip the top into ½ cup of powdered sugar. Place on a non-stick cookie sheet with the sugar side up. Bake for 12 to 15 minutes depending upon how crisp you like them. Serve warm.

Note: Ginger is great for combatting nausea. This is a good dish to prepare for a loved one.

Serves: 36
Prep Time: 0:20

Calories 109	Carbohydrate 25g	Carbohydrate 25g
Protein 1g	Fat 1g	Dietary Fiber 4g
	% Calories from fat 3%	

Key Lime Pie

1 cup Graham cracker crumbs	½ cup sugar
2 tablespoons unsalted butter	½ teaspoon vanilla extract
1 tablespoon water	2 cups nonfat yogurt
1 packet gelatin powder	1 tablespoon lime rind
6 tablespoons fresh lime juice	

Mix the Graham cracker crumbs with the butter and line an 8 inch baking pan. Dissolve the gelatin powder in the water and add the lime juice and sugar. Heat in a small saucepan until the sugar is dissolved. Allow to cool and add the yogurt and fresh grated lime rind. When beginning to thicken, place on top of the crumbs and leave to set. Garnish with sugared fresh lime or lemon rind. Serve chilled.

Note: Good source of Vitamin C, B2 and Calcium.

Serves: 6
Prep Time: 0:20
Stand Time: 1:00

Calories 253	Carbohydrate 35g	Cholesterol 12mg
Protein 18g	Fat 6g	Dietary Fiber 1g
	% Calories from fat 19%	

Peanut Butter Sesame Seed Bars

½ cup vanilla protein powder	½ cup honey
¾ cup skim dry milk	2 tablespoons warm water
1 cup dry oatmeal flakes	2 tablespoons sesame seeds
¾ cup low-fat peanut butter	

Combine all of the ingredients in a mixing bowl. Spray a 9 X 9 baking pan with oil and press the mixture into the pan. Refrigerate for at least 30 minutes before cutting into brownie shaped bars.

Note: Excellent source of Vitamin B6, B1, B2, Folate, Niacin and Zinc. Good source of Vitamin A, Calcium and Iron.

Serves: 12
Prep Time: 0:05
Stand Time: 0:30

Calories 143	Carbohydrate 25g	Cholesterol 1mg
Protein 9g	Fat 2g	Dietary Fiber 2g
	% Calories from fat 9%	

Cinnamon Apple Sauce

2 cups apple sauce
1 teaspoon cinnamon

For homemade apple sauce, wash, peel and core 1 pound of apples. Add piece of lemon and cook over low heat until soft. Blend and sweeten to taste. Add cinnamon.

Notes: You can also purchase ready made apple sauce for a quick and easy dessert. Baby food size is useful for single servings. Good source of Vitamin C.

Serving Size: 4
Prep Time: 0:20

Calories 68	Carbohydrate 18g	Cholesterol 0mg
Protein <1g	Fat <1g	Dietary Fiber 3g
	% Calories from fat 6%	

Pineapple Meringue Pie

1 cup pineapple chunks, light syrup
1 cup pineapple juice
1 tablespoon butter
1 tablespoon flour
1 egg yolk
½ cup sugar
2 egg whites

Preheat the oven to 350°F. Drain the pineapple chunks and retain the light syrup. Melt the butter in a sauce-pan and add the flour. Stir over a gentle heat for 2-3 minutes until a roux forms and the mixture comes away from the sides easily. Add the syrup and pineapple juice (total of one cup) and bring to a boil, stirring all the time. When the sauce is thickened, add the egg yolk and all of the pineapple chunks except one or two for decoration. Remove from the heat and pour into a greased 9" pie dish. Beat the egg whites until fluffy but not dry. Fold in the sugar and continue to beat until shiny and stiff. Spoon over the pineapple mixture and garnish with the left over pineapple chunks. Place in the oven for 3-4 minutes until the top has browned.

Serve hot.

Note: Excellent source of Vitamin C.
Serves: 6
Prep Time: 0:20

Calories 146	Carbohydrate 29g	Cholesterol 41mg
Protein 2.1g	Fat 3g	Dietary Fiber 1g
	% Calories from fat 17%	

Fresh Fruit Salad

- 1 apple, peeled and chopped
- 8 small seedless grapes, peeled
- 1 can mandarin oranges, light syrup
- 1 plum, chopped
- 1 nectarine, chopped
- ½ banana, peeled and sliced
- 1 pear, peeled and chopped
- 2 tablespoons lemon juice

Combine all of the ingredients in a mixing bowl. Chill in the refrigerator for at least one hour. Transfer to individual dessert dishes and serve garnished with tiny sprigs of mint or borage.

Notes: Excellent source of Vitamin C, A, B6 and Iron. Good source of Vitamin B1, B2 and Folic acid. For added 3 A's benefit (Antioxidant, Anticarcinogen and Anti-inflammatory) include the oils from the zest of the lemons as you squeeze them.
Serves: 4
Prep Time: 0:20
Stand Time: 1:00

Calories 320	Carbohydrate 82g	Cholesterol 0mg
Protein 4g	Fat 1g	Dietary Fiber 8g
	% Calories from fat 3%	

Fresh Peaches in Lemon Juice

- 6 fresh peaches, peeled and sliced
- 2 tablespoons sugar
- 2 lemons, juiced

Arrange peach slices in a serving dish and cover with the sugar and lemon juice. Leave for at least 2 hours in the refrigerator. The peaches will leach juice into the lemon juice and create a sweet sauce with the sugar. This is best served at room temperature after a main course of meat to cleanse the palate.

Note: Excellent source of Vitamin C. Good source of Vitamin A.
Serves: 4
Prep Time: 0:05
Stand Time: 2:00

Calories 91	Carbohydrate 26g	Cholesterol 0mg

Protein 2g | Fat <1g | Dietary Fiber 3g
% Calories from fat 2%

Pears in Red Wine

- 4 pears
- 3 cups red wine
- ¾ cup sugar
- ½ teaspoon cinnamon
- 1 cup water
- 2 tablespoons fresh lemon juice

Peel and core the pears. Cover with cold water and add the lemon juice to prevent them from turning brown. In a large saucepan place the red wine, sugar, cinnamon and water. Heat the mixture until the sugar is dissolved. Add the pears and simmer gently for 10-15 minutes until soft, turning them so they are evenly colored by the wine. Remove the pears when soft and place in a serving dish. Bring to the liquid to a boil and reduce by half. Coat the pears with the sauce and serve warm.

Note: Good source of Vitamin C.
Serves: 4
Prep Time: 0:20

Calories 373 | Carbohydrate 66g | Cholesterol 0mg
Protein 1g | Fat 1g | Dietary Fiber 4g
% Calories from fat 2%

Strawberry Delight

- 1 packet gelatin powder, dissolved in water
- 1 cup low fat yogurt with fruit
- ½ cup fresh sliced strawberries

Prepare the gelatin according to the instructions. When it begins to set, stir in the yogurt and strawberries. Pour into individual dessert dishes and refrigerate until set. Garnish with fresh strawberries and whipped cream.

Note: Excellent source of Calcium.
Serves: 4
Prep Time: 0:15
Standing Time: 2:00

Calories 143 | Carbohydrate 31g | Cholesterol 3mg
Protein 4g | Fat <1g | Dietary Fiber <1g
% Calories from fat 5%

Rhubarb and Cinnamon Pie

- 1 cup Graham cracker crumbs
- 2 tablespoons unsalted butter
- 1 pound fresh rhubarb
- ¼ cup sugar
- 2 tablespoons flour
- ½ teaspoon cinnamon
- 2 tablespoons cream cheese
- 1 tablespoon sour cream

Combine Graham cracker crumbs with melted butter and line 8 inch baking pan. Prepare rhubarb by washing, removing any blemished or coarse parts and then slicing and cutting into 1/2 inch pieces. Place rhubarb in pie crust. Mix sugar, flour, cream cheese and cinnamon and then spoon over the rhubarb. Bake in pre-heated oven at 425 degrees for 30 minutes. Allow to cool and serve with fresh, whipped cream garnished with a little cinnamon.

Note: Cinnamon is good for stabilizing blood sugar levels.
Serves: 6
Prep Time: 0:10
Baking Time: 0:30

Calories 166	Carbohydrate 25g	Cholesterol 14 mg
Protein 3 g	Fat 7 g	Dietary Fiber 2 g
	% Calories from fat 38%	

BEVERAGES AND SMOOTHIES

Aloha Delight

- 1 cup skim milk
- 2 tablespoons vanilla protein powder
- ½ teaspoon coconut extract
- ½ teaspoon pineapple extract
- 1 tablespoon orange juice
- 3 ice cubes

Combine ingredients in a blender and blend until smooth. Serve chilled, garnished with fresh pineapple and a sprig of mint.

Note: Excellent source of Vitamin C, B1, B2, Calcium and Iron. Good source of Vitamin A and B6.
Serves: 1
Prep Time: 0:05

Calories 186	Carbohydrate 24g	Cholesterol 4mg
Protein 17g	Fat 1g	Dietary Fiber 3g
	% Calories from fat 6%	

Apple Pie Smoothie

- 2 tablespoons vanilla protein powder
- ¼ cup apples
- a dash nutmeg
- ½ teaspoon cinnamon
- 1 cup skim milk
- 3 ice cubes

Blend all ingredients together and serve chilled.

Note: Excellent source of Vitamin C, B6, B12, B1, B2, Folate, Calcium, Iron and Zinc. Good source of Vitamin A.

Serves: 1
Prep Time: 0:10

Calories 184	Carbohydrate 27g	Cholesterol 4mg
Protein 16g	Fat 1g	Dietary Fiber 4g
	% Calories from fat 6%	

Banana Fruit Smoothie

- 2 tablespoons vanilla protein powder
- 4 ounces nonfat yogurt
- 4 fluid ounces water
- ½ cup frozen peaches
- ½ medium banana
- 3 ice cubes

Blend all ingredients and serve chilled, garnished with a slice of banana.

Note: Excellent source of Vitamin C, B6, B1, B2, Iron and Zinc. Good source of Calcium.

Serves: 1
Prep Time: 0:05

Calories 310	Carbohydrate 62g	Cholesterol 2mg
Protein 16g	Fat 1g	Dietary Fiber 6g
	% Calories from fat 3%	

Black Forest Smoothie

- 2 tablespoons chocolate protein powder
- ½ teaspoon black walnut extract
- 8 fluid ounces skim milk
- ½ banana
- 4 ice cubes

Combine ingredients in a blender and serve chilled garnished with chocolate sprinkles.

Notes: Excellent source of Vitamin C, B6, B12, B1, B2, Calcium and Zinc. Good source of Vitamin A and Iron.

Serves: 1
Prep Time: 0:05

Calories 175	Carbohydrate 26g	Cholesterol 9mg
Protein 16g	Fat 1g	Dietary Fiber 16g
	% Calories from fat 5%	

Cappuccino Smoothie

- 2 tablespoons chocolate protein powder
- 4 ounces vanilla frozen yogurt
- 1 tablespoon instant coffee
- 3 ice cubes
- 4 fluid ounces skim milk

Place all ingredients in a blender and mix until smooth. Garnish with chocolate coffee bean.

Note: Excellent source of Vitamin B12, B2 and Calcium.

Serves: 1

Prep Time: 0:05

Calories 196	Carbohydrate 28g	Cholesterol 4mg
Protein 19g	Fat 1g	Dietary Fiber 0g
	% Calories from fat 4%	

Extra Chocolatey Smoothie

- 1 cup skim milk
- 2 tablespoons chocolate protein powder
- ¼ teaspoon chocolate syrup
- 1 teaspoon Hershey's cocoa
- ¼ teaspoon vanilla extract
- 3 ice cubes

Combine all the ingredients in a blender and blend until smooth. Serve chilled. Top with sprinkles.
Note: Excellent source of Vitamin B12, B2 and Calcium. Good source of Vitamin A. Optional addition: 1 teaspoon instant coffee.

Serves: 1

Prep Time: 0:05

Calories 184	Carbohydrate 28g	Cholesterol 9mg
Protein 17g	Fat 1g	Dietary Fiber 4g
	% Calories from fat 5%	

Fruit-Juicy Smoothie

- 2 tablespoons berry protein powder
- 8 fluid ounces cranberry juice
- 4 strawberries
- 3 ice cubes

Combine ingredients in a blender and serve chilled, garnished with a strawberry.

Note: Excellent source of Vitamin C, B6, B1, B2, Iron and Zinc. Good source of Calcium.

Serves: 1

Prep Time: 0:05

Calories 125	Carbohydrate 21g	Cholesterol 0mg
Protein 8g	Fat 1g	Dietary Fiber 3g
	% Calories from fat 7%	

Kiwi Quencher

- 2 tablespoons vanilla protein powder
- 8 fluid ounces water
- 1 kiwi fruit
- ½ banana
- 3 ice cubes
- 2 drops green chartreuse

Combine ingredients in a blender. Serve chilled with a slice of kiwi fruit as garnish.

Note: Excellent source of Vitamin C, B6, B2, Iron and Zinc. Good source of Vitamin B1.

Serves: 1

Prep Time: 0:05

Calories 80	Carbohydrate 10g	Cholesterol 0mg
Protein 8g	Fat <1g	Dietary Fiber 3g
	% Calories from fat 7%	

Mango Special

- 2 cups mangos diced
- 2 cups orange juice
- 2 tablespoons sugar
- ¼ cup lime juice
- ¼ cup lemon juice
- 2 cups water
- 3 ice cubes

Combine the ingredients in a blender. Strain and serve in a pitcher either for breakfast or as a non-alcoholic cocktail. This is excellent with champagne.

Note: Excellent source of Vitamin C and A. Good source of Folate.

Serves: 8

Prep Time: 0:10

Calories 70	Carbohydrate 18g	Cholesterol 0mg
Protein 1g	Fat 3g	Dietary Fiber 1g
	% Calories from Fat 3%	

Orange Blossom Smoothie

- 2 tablespoons vanilla protein powder
- ½ teaspoon orange extract
- 8 fluid ounces skim milk
- ½ orange
- 3 ice cubes

Combine ingredients in a blender and serve chilled, garnished with a slice of orange.

Note: Excellent source of Vitamin C, B6, B12, B1, B2, Calcium, Iron and Zinc. Good source of Vitamin A.

Serves: 1

Prep Time: 0:05

Calories 168	Carbohydrate 22g	Cholesterol 4mg
Protein 16g	Fat 1g	Dietary Fiber 3g
	% Calories from fat 6%	

Passionate Papaya Smoothie

- 2 tablespoons vanilla protein powder
- ½ papaya
- 8 fluid ounces apple juice
- a dash cinnamon

Blend together and serve chilled. Garnish with sprig of mint or borage.

Note: Excellent source of Vitamin C, B6, B1, B2, Folate, Iron and Zinc. Good source of Vitamin A.

Serves: 1
Prep Time: 0:05

Calories 256	Carbohydrate 54g	Cholesterol 0mg
Protein 10g	Fat 1g	Dietary Fiber 6g
	% Calories from fat 4%	

Peach Milk Smoothie

2 tablespoons vanilla protein powder
8 fluid ounces skim milk
1 teaspoon peach brandy extract (optional)
½ fresh peach
3 ice cubes

Combine ingredients in a blender and serve chilled, garnished with a slice of peach.

Note: Excellent source of Vitamin C, B6, B12, B1, B2, Calcium, Iron and Zinc. Good source of Vitamin A.

Serves: 1
Prep Time: 0:05

Calories 165	Carbohydrate 22g	Cholesterol 4mg
Protein 16g	Fat 1g	Dietary Fiber 3g
	% Calories from fat 6%	

Prune Smoothie

2 tablespoons vanilla protein powder
8 fluid ounces prune juice

Blend. Serve chilled.

Note: Excellent source of Vitamin C, B6, B1, B2, Iron and Zinc. Good source of Niacin.

Serves: 1
Prep Time: 0:05

Calories 216	Carbohydrate 44g	Cholesterol 0mg
Protein 9g	Fat 1g	Dietary Fiber 4g
	% Calories from fat 3%	

Raspberry RazMaTaz

2 tablespoons chocolate protein powder
8 fluid ounces water
1 cup raspberries, fresh or frozen
½ banana
3 ice cubes

Combine all ingredients in a blender. Serve chilled, garnished with fresh raspberries and a sprig of mint or borage.

Note: Excellent source of Vitamin C and Folate.
Serves: 1
Prep Time: 0:05

Calories 162	Carbohydrate 32g	Cholesterol 5mg
Protein 9g	Fat <1g	Dietary Fiber 7g
	% Calories from fat 5%	

Soda Fountain Shake

- 2 tablespoons vanilla protein powder
- 5 fluid ounces skim milk
- 3 fluid ounces seltzer water
- ½ banana
- 3 ice cubes

Blend together and serve chilled. Banana may be substituted with peach. Garnish with a slice of banana.

Note: Excellent source of Vitamin C, B6, B1, B2, Calcium, Iron and Zinc.
Serves: 1
Prep Time: 0:05

Calories 133	Carbohydrate 18g	Cholesterol 2mg
Protein 13g	Fat 1g	Dietary Fiber 3g
	% Calories from fat 6%	

Spicy Tomato Juice

- 2 cups tomato juice
- 1 teaspoon Tabasco sauce
- 1 teaspoon fresh lemon juice
- 2 stalks celery
- a pinch salt
- a pinch sugar

Combine all the ingredients in a jug. Chill for 30 minutes and serve garnished with celery stalks.

Note: Excellent source of Vitamin A, C, Folate. Good source of Vitamin B1 and Niacin.

Serves: 2
Prep Time: 0:10

Calories 133	Carbohydrate 18g	Cholesterol 0mg
Protein 13g	Fat 1g	Dietary Fiber 3g
	% Calories from fat 6%	

Strawberry Daiquiri

- 6 fluid ounces rum
- ½ cup fresh lime juice
- 2 tablespoons sugar
- 4 cups strawberries
- 6 ice cubes

Combine rum, lime juice, sugar and ice cubes in a blender. Add the strawberries after the sugar has dissolved and continue to blend at high speed until the mixture is smooth. Serve with sugar around the rim of each glass.

Note: Excellent source of Vitamin C. Good source of Folate.

Serves: 4
Prep Time: 0:10

Calories 173	Carbohydrate 20g	Cholesterol 0mg
Protein 1g	Fat 1g	Dietary Fiber 4g
	% Calories from fat 6%	

Strawberry Sensation

- 2 tablespoons strawberry protein powder
- 8 fluid ounces water
- 1 cup strawberries
- 1 apricot
- 3 ice cubes

Combine all ingredients in a blender. Garnish with a strawberry and sprig of fresh mint.

Note: Excellent source of Vitamin C, B6, B1, B2, Iron and Zinc. Good source of Folate and Calcium.

Serves: 1
Prep Time: 0:05

Calories 124	Carbohydrate 21g	Cholesterol 0mg
Protein 9g	Fat 2g	Dietary Fiber 6g
	% Calories from fat 11%	

Vanilla Shake

- 2 tablespoons vanilla protein powder
- 6 fluid ounces skim milk
- 3 ice cubes
- 4 ounces nonfat yogurt

Blend all ingredients together. Serve chilled, garnished with fresh fruit.

Note: Excellent source of Vitamin B6, B12, B2, Calcium and Zinc. Good source of Vitamin C, B1 and Iron.

Serves: 1
Prep Time: 0:05

Calories 228	Carbohydrate 31g	Cholesterol 6mg
Protein 23g	Fat 1g	Dietary Fiber 3g
	% Calories from fat 5%	

Wild Berry-Orange Smoothie

2	tablespoons berry protein powder	4	strawberries
8	fluid ounces orange juice	3	ice cubes

Combine all ingredients in a blender and serve chilled, garnished with a fresh strawberry.

Notes: Excellent source of Vitamin C, B6, B1, B2, Folate, Iron and Zinc. Good source of Vitamin A and Calcium.

Serves: 1
Prep Time: 0:05

Calories 192	Carbohydrate 36g	Cholesterol 0mg
Protein 10g	Fat 2g	Dietary Fiber 3g
	% Calories from fat 7%	

RECIPE INDEX

Appetizers

Soups and Broths

Beans, Pasta and Rice

Fish

Chicken

Vegetables and Vegetarian Dishes

Desserts and Comfort Foods

Beverages and Smoothies

HANDBOOK TEXT INDEX

BIBLIOGRAPHY and FURTHER READING

Clinical Oncology, 3rd Edtion. Editors Raymond, E. Lenhard, J. et al. American Cancer Society, 2004.
Nutrition for the Chemotherapy Patient, Janet Ramstack, DrPH and Ernest H. Rosenbaum, MD. Bull Publishing, 1990.
Nutritional Oncology, 2nd Edition. Editors., Blackburn, G. Vay Liang W. Go., Milner, J., and D. Heber. Academic Press, 2006.
The Omega Plan, Artemis Simopoulos, MD and Jo Robinson. Harper Collins, 1998.
The Wellness Community Guide to Fighting for Recovery from Cancer,
Harold H. Benjamin, PhD. Tarcher Putnam, 1995.
Radiation Therapy and You; a guide to self help during treatment. National Cancer Institute pub #92-2227
Chemotherapy and You. National Cancer Institute pub #94-1136
Eating Hints for Cancer Patients; before, during and after treatment. National Cancer Institute pub #99-2079
Trease & Evans' Pharmacognosy. By W.C. Evans. W.B.Saunders, 2002.
The Strang Cancer Prevention Center Cookbook by L. Pensiero, S. Oliveria and
M. Osborne, MD. Dutton 1998, and paperback 2004.
Nutrition and physical activity during and after cancer treatment: an American Cancer Society guide for informed choices. CA Cancer J Clin. 2003 Sep-Oct; 53(5):268-91. Brown JK, Byers T, Doyle C, Coumeya KS, Demark-Wahnefried W, Kushi LH, McTieman A, Rock CL, Aziz N, Bloch AS, Eldridge B, Hamilton K, Katzin C, Koonce A, Main J, Mobley C, Morra ME, Pierce MS, Sawyer KA; American Cancer Society.

Links

http://cissecure.nci.nih.gov/hcipubs to order free NCI publications
www.eatright.org The American Dietetic Association website for nutrition information and to find a local dietitian.
www.cancer.org The American Cancer Society.
www.cert-nutrition.org The Certification board of Nutrition Specialists for information about Certified Nutrition Specialists (CNS). CBNS is affiliated with American College of Nutrition www.am-coll-nutr.org which publishes the Journal of the American College of Nutrition.
www.wellness-community.org The Wellness Community for information about local support groups, seminars and activities

NOTES